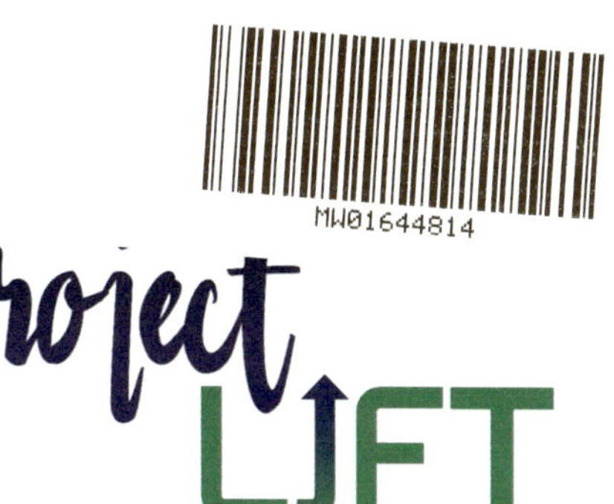

A PREVENTION AND SOCIAL JUSTICE AGENCY

RESOURCE DIRECTORY FOR MEN

CUYAHOGA COUNTY

SUMMER 2025

DID YOU KNOW?

Black males have some of the poorest social health determinants, such as mental health crises, homelessness, incarceration, and premature death resulting from homicide, suicide, and physical illness.

These experiences not only result in the individual's instability but have a rippling impact within their families and communities.

Disrupting these outcomes requires an intentional investment in raising awareness of behavioral health treatment and prevention resources and services.

Collectively, we can create a healthier, responsive, and more inclusive healthcare system and services.

#preventionworks #recoveryispossible #mentalhealthmatters

Mental Health Check-In

If you are experiencing any of the symptoms below, consider contacting a behavioral health professional today!

Ask yourself how you're feeling

The COVID-19 pandemic is an event that has never been experienced in our lifetime bringing with it a host of potentially new emotions, physical symptoms, and mental health issues.

Be Aware of Signs & Symptoms

Signs & Symptoms of Anxiety

Occasional anxiety is an expected part of life. But anxiety disorders involve more than temporary worry or fear.

- Feeling restless, wound-up, or on-edge
- Being easily fatigued
- Having difficulty concentrating; mind going blank
- Difficulty controlling feelings of worry

Signs & Symptoms of Depression

If you have been experiencing some of the following signs and symptoms most of the day, nearly every day, for at least two weeks, you may be suffering from depression:

- Irritability
- Feelings of guilt, worthlessness, or helplessness
- Difficulty concentrating, remembering, or making decisions
- Aches or pains, headaches, cramps, or digestive problems without a clear physical cause and/or that do not ease even with treatment

Care for Yourself & Others

Make sure **self-care** remains a priority.

If you need support, are feeling lonely and overwhelmed with emotions such as sadness, depression, anxiety, or feel like you want to harm yourself or someone else, call 911 or the 988.

Adapted from Ohio Department of Mental Health and Addiction Services www.mha.ohio.gov

What is Grief?

Experiencing loss is natural and normal and begins in our childhood. The loss may have been a person, item, pet, and even an idea or dream you may have had for yourself. Because loss is quite common, we often fail to stop and grieve the loss to allow healing.

Instead, we try to push forward and get through it, believing time heals all wounds.

For many Black males, loss has become a part of everyday life. Far too many are dealing with traumatic and persistent loss of safety, loved ones, and dreams. This chronic experience can have a negative impact on your mood, beliefs, actions, and even your self-worth. It can create a feeling of powerlessness and helplessness, resulting in depression, anxiety, and even aggressive behaviors.

Many Black males are hurting from loss and don't know how to access help.

What's worse, many believe there is no help or that people will not understand.

You do not have to do this alone.

Your life matters and so does your healing and joy!

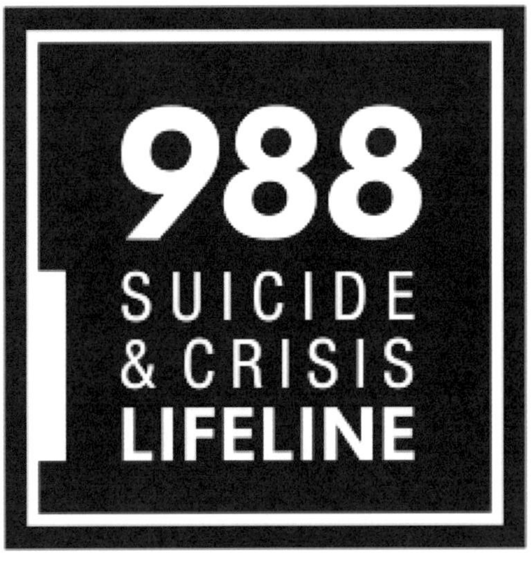

Suicide is a major public health concern in Ohio. Suicide is complicated and tragic, but it is often preventable.

Don't hesitate to obtain the support your need!

Project LIFT Services 501c3 is a prevention and social justice agency serving males 14 and older. We target the needs of Black teens and fathers most at-risk for homelessness, economic instability, and incarceration who live within Cuyahoga County. Project LIFT provides a continuum of services including linkage and referral to community resources, psychoeducational groups to build parenting skills, as well as, counseling. Project LIFT utilizes evidence-based practices to improve coping skills, address trauma experiences, engage in academic/vocational goal planning, and enhance recovery and prevention.

In addition to serving clients directly, we offer continuing education for professionals seeking CEU's or those who want to build their knowledge and skills. Our clinical and human service training include cultural inclusivity, diagnosing, with practical strategies to engage clients with complex trauma histories.

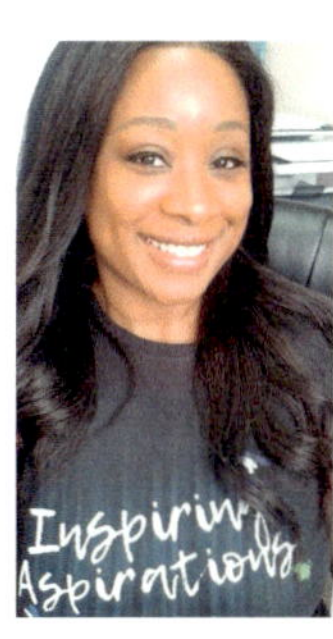

"I wanted to provide a user-friendly guide for young men ages 14 and up, with resources that specifically addresses their needs. I am hopeful this guide will help young men obtain the support they need to thrive!

LaToya Logan, MSSA LISW-S ABD

Chief Executive Officer and Founder

Meet the Team

Keith Brown Jr.

Sylvia Lewis

Corryn Freeman-Wells

Crystal Sledge

Lakiesha Smith

Tanyell Logan

Laurese Glover

La'Dell Thedford

Camellia Dabney

Destiny Curlee

Faizah Rahman

Bianca Scarbrough

4415 Euclid Ave Ste. 315 Cleveland, OH 44103

(216) 465-2000 (T) (216) 916-4803 (F)

www.projectliftservices.org

Table of Contents

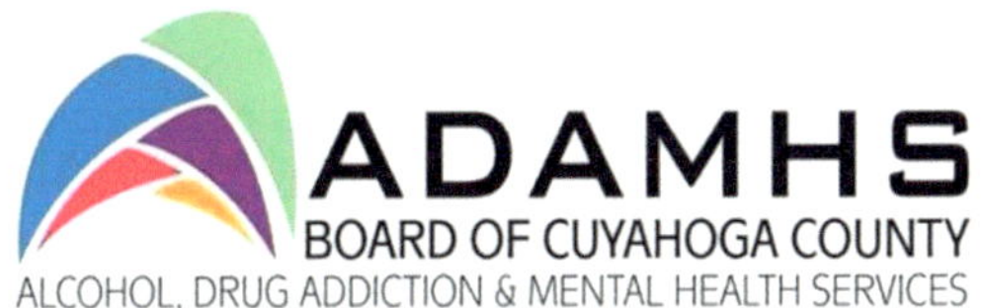

The ADAMHS Board mission is to enhance the quality of life for our community through a commitment to excellence in mental health and addiction prevention, treatment and recovery services coordinated through a person-centered network of community supports. Mental health, addiction, prevention, treatment and recovery services will be available and accessible for every county resident in need and the ADAMHS Board will provide a preeminent, seamless and integrated system of care.

24/7 Hotline : 216-623-6888

(216) 241-3400

adamhscc.org

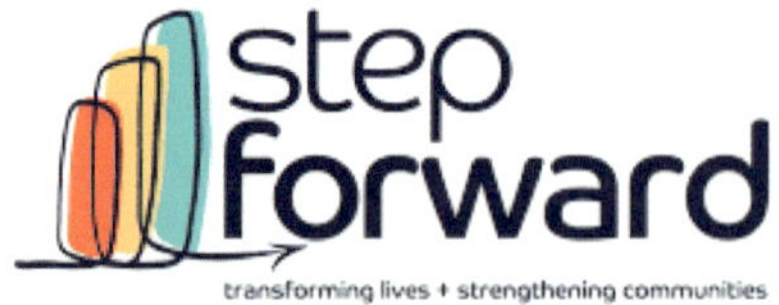

- **Phone**: 216-696-9077
- **Address**: 1801 Superior Ave., Ste 400, Cleveland, OH 44114
- **Messenger on website**
- **Offers**: Head Start, , energy assistance, personal and professional development, housing assistance, financial assistance
- **Website**: stepforwardtoday.org

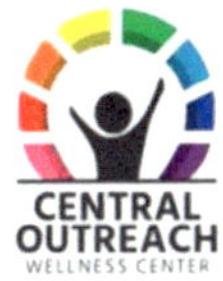

CENTRAL OUTREACH WELLNESS CENTER

Inclusive healthcare with dignity and respect.

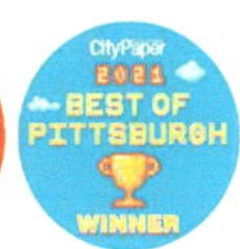

Our mission is to promote wellness in our community by fostering our patient's whole self. Our focus is on culturally competent care by striving to understand what our client's needs are and how we can treat them holistically.

We provide the following services: HIV & PrEP, HEP C testing and cure, STD 0testing, cosmetic services, medical, and so much more!

2040 Lee Road, Cleveland Heights, Cleveland, OH 44118

centraloutreach.com

216-350-1000

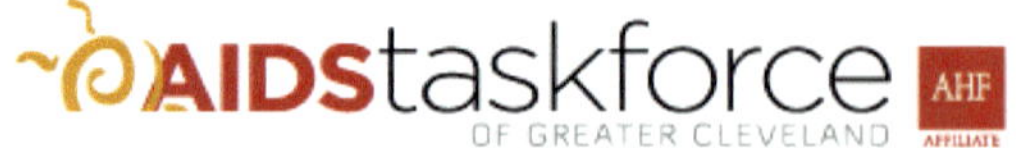

Founded in 1983, The AIDS Taskforce of Greater Cleveland (ATGC) is the oldest and largest AIDS Service Organization (ASO) in Ohio. We annually provide social and medical services to nearly 1,000 clients living with HIV and prevention services to over 25,000 at greatest risk for acquiring the virus that causes AIDS. Our organization provides a coordinated and collaborative response to HIV/AIDS epidemic affecting Northeast Ohio.

first tee
cleveland

First Tee - Cleveland represents a moral and long term commitment to the children of our city. While using recreation, it goes far beyond recreation. Throughout the program there is a seamless integration of life skills. Further, the operation of a golf course and a continuing collaborative relationship between the Cleveland Metroparks, the City of Cleveland, and First Tee - Cleveland will provide additional skill training and employment opportunities.

3883 Washington Park Blvd., Newburgh Heights, OH 44105

plopresti@FirstTeeCleveland.org

216-641-7799

firstteecleveland.org

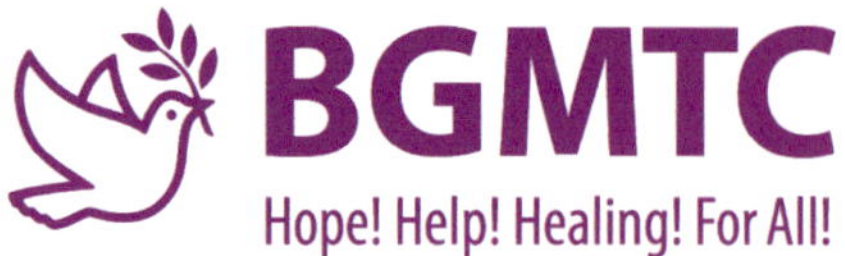

The Brenda Glass Multipurpose Trauma Center is a nonprofit service organization in Cleveland that provides professional counseling and support services to victims of crime and violence. We offer an array of mental health services, spiritual counseling, case management, and linkage to safe shelter to Cuyahoga County residents who have been impacted by crime, physical violence, or sexual assault.

440-836-2576

Bglass@brendaglasstraumacenter.org

Services available 24/7

brendaglasstraumacenter.org

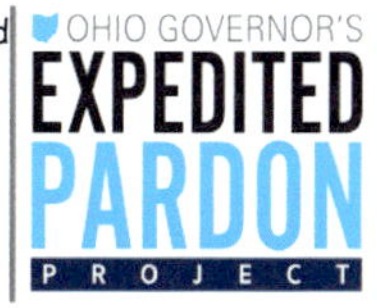

The Expedited Pardon Project was launched by Governor DeWine to help citizens move quickly through the pardon process.

First applicants must fill out the intake paperwork and submit it to the Project Team.

The Project Team will determine the applicant's eligibility (meets all requirements and has no disqualifying offenses). The Project Team will then help the applicant fill out and submit the Pardon Application to the Ohio Parole Board.

The Ohio Parole Board then sends the application and makes a recommendation to the Ohio Governor and the Governor makes the final decision on whether to pardon or not.

Contact Project LIFT Services at (216) 465-2000 to find out

how we can help you meet eligibility criteria!

Access the application and more at www.ohiopardonproject.org

LIFTED X Barbershop

We are proud to partner with the following barbershops:

- Epic - 11204 Lorain Ave.
- Diamond Cuts - 5139 Superior
- 2nd Round Knockouts - 15732 Lorain Ave.
- Earle's - 12603 Buckeye Rd.
- Classic Clippers - 9718 Buckeye
- Perfect Blend - 20117 Harvard
- Station Six - 12401 Larchmere
- Polished Professionals - 12501 Larchmere

Each of our barbershop partners are provided with resources monthly including:

- Wellness Kits with hygiene items, stress relief items, and more
- Resource Directory of Cuyahoga County resources
- Tip cards covering mental health, substance use, suicide prevention, healthy relationships, etc....
- Free blood pressure, blood sugar, and nutritional screenings
- Monthly Health Pop ups!

We would like to say thank you to all our barbers for allowing us to host our Health pop ups and wellness talks at their shops. We are honored to partner with a key part of the Black community to provide awareness, education, and resources. Thank you for the opportunity to assist you all in creating a safe and inclusive space for Black males to be themselves and learn about their wellness.
We are beyond grateful and we will see you at the next Health pop up!

Special Thanks to

- James @ Platinum Stylez
- Jarmaine @ Second Round Knockout
- Lee @ Classic Clippers
- Mook @ Diamond Cut
- Da'John @ Epic
- JB and Lathan @ Polished Professionals
- Marcus @Station six
- Jason @ First Draft Pick 2

Crisis Support: 24/7 

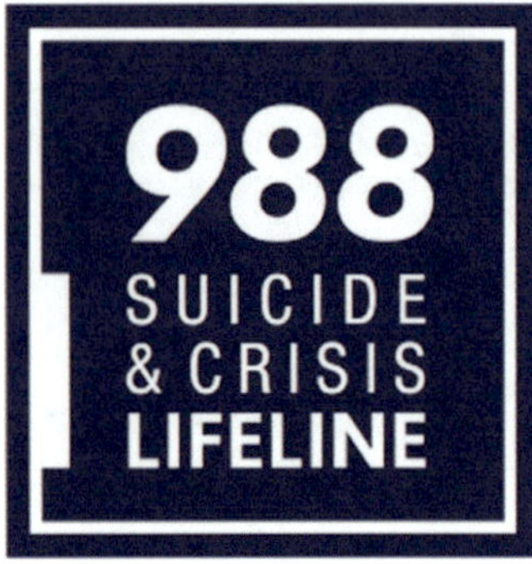

Suicide is a major public health concern in Ohio. Suicide is complicated and tragic, but it is often preventable.

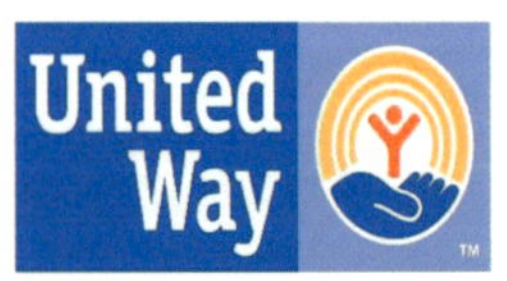

2-1-1 HelpLink is a free and confidential 24/7 helpline that connects people in need with more than 2,500 area agencies to ensure they receive essential resources such as utility, food, and shelter assistance.

24/7 Crisis Hotline: 2-1-1

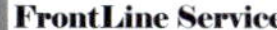

FrontLine Service

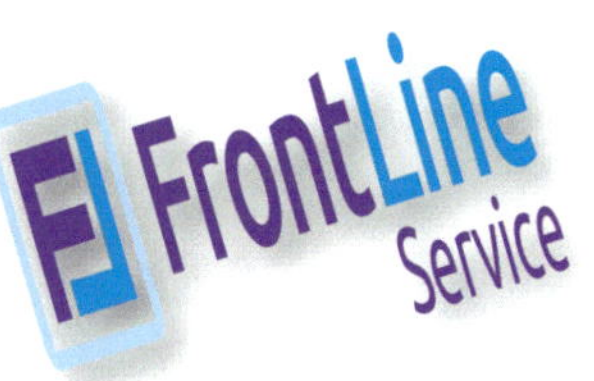

If you need support we are available 24 hours a day, 7 days a week. This is a judge-free space. We listen to you and keep you safe. We help you explore your feelings, thoughts, and opinions about whatever it is that may be causing you distress. We offer information about local resources and are with you the entire way.

24/7 Crisis Hotline: 216-623-6888

24/7 Text Hotline: Text '4Hope' to 741741

Chat online: frontlineservice.org

The Veterans Crisis Line is a free, confidential resource that's available to anyone, even if you're not registered with VA or enrolled in VA health care. The caring, qualified responders at the Veterans Crisis Line are specially trained and experienced in helping Veterans of all ages and circumstances.

24/7 Crisis Line: 988 Press 1

24/7 Text Line: 838255

Chat online: veteranscrisisline.net/

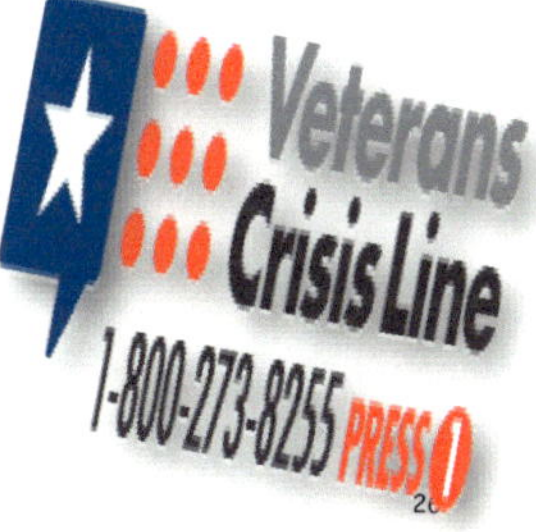

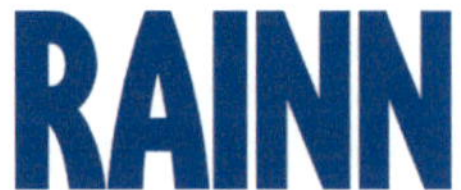

RAINN (Rape, Abuse & Incest National Network) is the nation's largest anti-sexual violence organization. RAINN created and operates the National Sexual Assault Hotline in partnership with more than 1,000 local sexual assault service providers across the country and operates the DoD Safe Helpline for the Department of Defense. RAINN also carries out programs to prevent sexual violence, help survivors, and ensure that perpetrators are brought to justice.

24/7 Crisis Hotline: 800-656-4673

Chat online: online.rainn.org

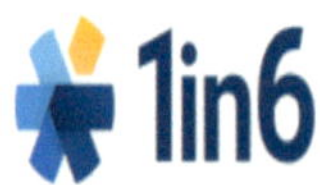

The mission of **1in6** is to help men who have had unwanted or abusive sexual experiences live healthier, happier lives. Our mission also includes serving family members, friends, partners, and service providers by providing information and support resources on the web and in the community.

Chat online: 1in6.org/helpline/

24/7 Crisis line: 1-800-656-4673

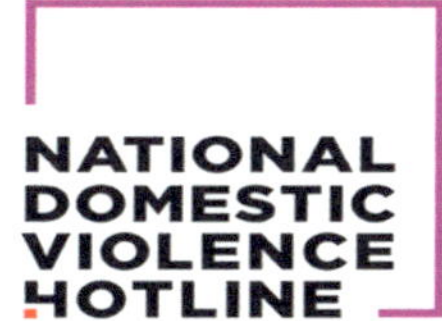

National Domestic Violence Hotline provides essential tools and support to help survivors of domestic violence so they can live their lives free of abuse. Contacts to The Hotline can expect highly-trained, expert advocates to offer free, confidential, and compassionate support, crisis intervention information, education, and referral services in over 200 languages.

24/7 Crisis hotline: 1-800-799-7233
24/7 Crisis hotline TTY: 1-800-787-3224
Text "START" to 88788
Chat line: thehotline.org/#

Polaris assists thousands of victims and survivors through the U.S. National Human Trafficking Hotline, helped ensure countless traffickers were held accountable and built the largest known U.S. data set on actual trafficking experiences. With the guidance of survivors, we use that data to improve the way trafficking is identified, how victims and survivors are assisted, and how communities, businesses and governments can prevent human trafficking by transforming the underlying inequities and oppressions that make it possible.

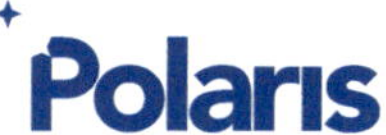

24/7 Crisis hotline: 1-888-373-7888
24/7 Text hotline: 'BEFREE' 233733
Online chat: humantraffickinghotline.org

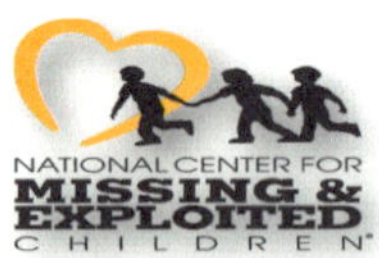

The National Center for Missing & Exploited Children is a private, non-profit 501(c)(3) corporation whose mission is to help find missing children, reduce child sexual exploitation, and prevent child victimization. NCMEC works with families, victims, private industry, law enforcement, and the public to assist with preventing child abductions, recovering missing children, and providing services to deter and combat child sexual exploitation.

24/7 Crisis hotline: 800-843-5678

Online reporting: cybertipline.org

Safe School Helpline®

The Helpline is a 24/7 communication service that empowers school administrators to make proactive decisions as well as creating responsibilities for students, parents and community members to share in the maintenance of a safe learning environment. We provide children with the opportunity to anonymously report wrongdoing, bullying, and negative issues that would impede the learning process.

24/7 Crisis hotline: 1-800-418-6423 ext.359

24/7 Crisis hotline (Cleveland Metropolitan School District Only): 216-771-7233

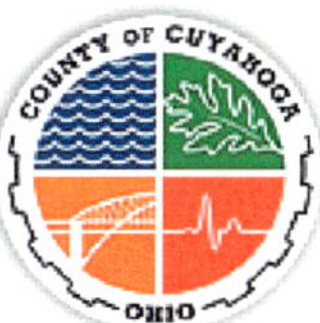

DCFS works to assure children at risk of abuse and neglect are protected and nurtured within a family and with the support of the community. Safety, permanency, and well-being are the goals for every child and family we encounter. Employees investigate allegations, assess child safety, and risk contributors, and help stabilize families that have been weakened through poverty, illness or crisis. We help achieve permanency through reunification, legal custody, or adoption.

24/7 Crisis hotline: 216-696-5437
Email: protecting-cuyahoga-kids@jfs.ohio.gov
Online report: cuyahogacounty.us/child-abuse-and-neglect

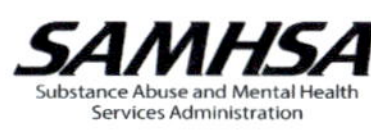

SAMHSA's National Helpline is a confidential, free, 24-hour-a-day, 365-day-a-year, information service, in English and Spanish, for individuals and family members facing mental and/or substance use disorders. This service provides referrals to local treatment facilities, support groups, and community-based organizations. Callers can also order free publications and other information.

24/7 Crisis hotline: 1-800-662-4357

24/7 TTY Crisis hotline: 1-800-487-4889

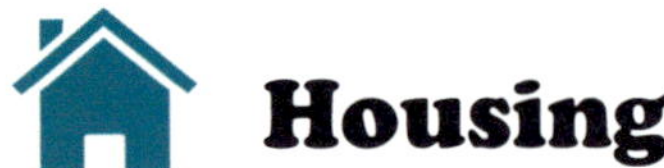

A Place 4 Me

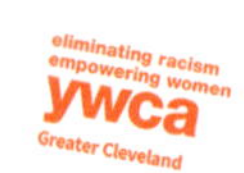

- **Phone**: 216-329-4001
- **Address**: 4100 Franklin Blvd. Cleveland, OH 44113
- **Email**: sjones@ywcacleveland.org
- **Offers**: Prevents youth homelessness, support services to youth 18-26, connects youth to resources
- **Website**: ywcaofcleveland.org/end-homelessness/a-place-4-me

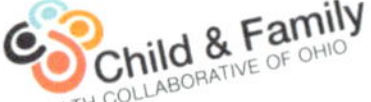

Bridges

- **Phone**: 614-461-0014 ext.20
- **Address**: 2600 Corporate Exchange Drive Ste. 180, Columbus, OH 43231
- **Messenger on website**
- **Offers**: Stable housing for those aging out of foster care, preventing homelessness, career readiness, job search assistance
- **Website**: cfhcohio.org/bridges-program

Cleveland Christian Home

- **Phone**: 216-416-4277
- **Address**: 11401 Lorain Ave., Cleveland, OH 44111
- **Email**: info@cchome.org
- **Offers**: Residential treatment up to 30 males ages 6-17, shelter, family preservation services, crisis intervention programs, family reunification, school-based programming, school counseling
- **Website**: cchome.org

Front Steps Housing and Services

- **Phone**: 216-781-2550
- **Address**: 2554 W 25th St., Cleveland, OH 44113
- **Email**: info@frontstepsservices.org
- **Offers**: Housing, independent living preparation, financial literacy, family reunification, peer support, case management, therapy, substance abuse services, workforce readiness workshops
- **Website**: frontstepsservices.org

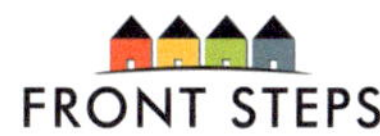

Joseph and Mary's Home

❖ **Phone**: 216-685-1551

❖ **Address**: 2412 Community College Ave., Cleveland, OH 44115

❖ **Email**: info@jmhome.org

❖ **Offers**: Shelter, medical respite, developing life skills programs

❖ **Website**: jmhome.org

Frontline Service

❖ **Phone**: 216-623-6555

❖ **Address**: 1744 Payne Ave., Cleveland, OH 44114

❖ **Messenger and Crisis Chat available on website**

❖ **Offers**: street outreach, emergency housing, support services, permanent supportive housing

❖ **Website**: frontlineservice.org

StandUp for Kids

❖ **Phone**:

216-820-3396

❖ **Email**:
cleveland@
standupforkids.
org

❖ **Offers:** Street outreach, supplies delivery, resource connection, outreach centers

❖ **Website**:
standupforkids.
org/cleveland

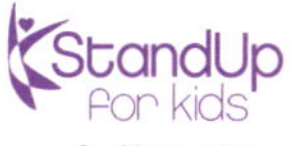

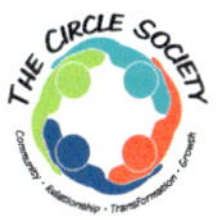

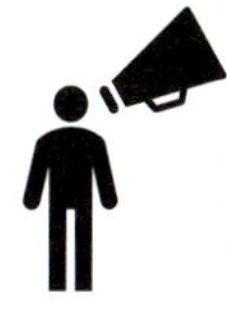

The Circle Society

❖ **Phone**:
216-206-7858

❖ **Address**:
12200 Fairhill Rd., Ste. C257, Cleveland, OH 44120

❖ **Email**:
info@
thecirclesociety.
org

❖ **Offers:** Personal development, life coaching, housing for children who aged out of the foster care system and aged individuals

❖ **Website**:
thecirclesociety.
org

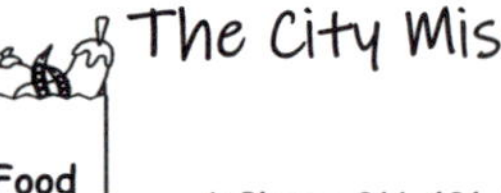

The City Mission

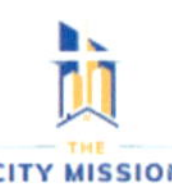

- **Phone**: 216-431-3510
- **Address**: 5310 Carnegie Ave., Cleveland, OH 44103
- **Messenger on Website**
- **Offers**: Shelter, emergency food assistance, case management, therapy, support groups
- **Website**: thecitymission.org

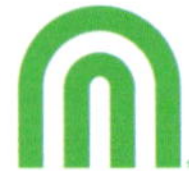

CHN Housing Partners

- **Phone**: 216-574-7100
- **Address**: 2999 Payne Ave., Suite 134, Cleveland, OH 44114
- **Email**: help@chnhousingpartners.org
- **Offers**: rental assistance, homebuyer assistance and programs, housing and apartments, rent to own programs, mortgage assistance
- **Website**: chnhousingpartners.org

Mental and Behavioral Health

Ascension Counseling and Therapy Services, LTD.

- **Phone**: 833-254-3278
- **Email**: intake@ascensioncounseling.com
- **Address**: 24100 Chagrin Blvd Suite 125, Beachwood, OH 44122
- **Offers**: Therapy, counseling, couples counseling, EMDR therapy, medication management, wellness services
- **Website**: ascensioncounseling.com

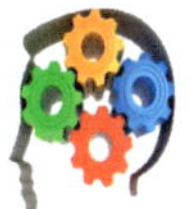

Cleveland Center for Cognitive Therapy

- **Phone**: 216-831-2500
- **Address**: 24400 Highpoint Rd., Ste. 9, Beachwood, OH 44122
- **Messenger on website**
- **Offers**: Counseling, therapy, training for professionals
- **Website**: clevelandcognitivetherapy.com

Carrington

- **Phone**: 216-268-2400
- **Address**: 2114 Noble Rd., Cleveland, OH 44112
- **Email**: referral@ carringtonkids.org
- **Offers**: Residential treatment, therapy, drug and alcohol treatment, psychiatric care, religious services, educational services
- **Website**: carringtonbh.org

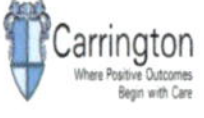

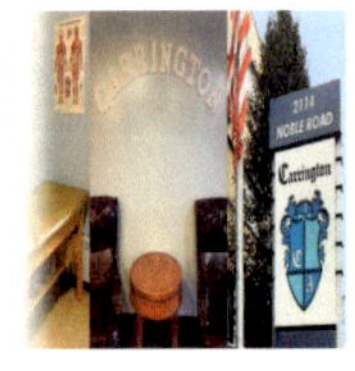

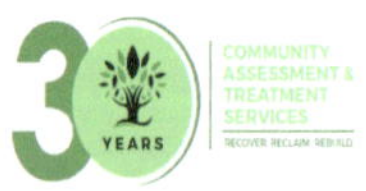

Community Assessment and Treatment Services

- **Phone**: 216-441-0200
- **Address**: 8411 Broadway Ave., Cleveland, OH 44105
- **Messenger on Website**
- **Offers**: Residential treatment, outpatient services, counseling, case management

Website: communityassessment.org

Community Behavioral Health Center

- **Phone**: 216-831-1494
- **Address**: 3690 Orange Place, Ste. 320, Beachwood, OH 44122
- **Email**: info@cbhcweb.com
- **Offers**: Psychiatric services, medication management, counseling, case management
- **Website**: cbhctr.com

Crossroads Health

- **Phone**: 440-255-1700
- **Address**: Multiple locations: Mentor, Painesville, Willoughby,
- **Messenger on Website**
- **Offers**: Psychiatry and medication management, counseling and therapy), school counseling, primary care, early childhood services, addiction recovery and treatment, criminal justice services
- **Website**: crossroadshealth.org

Daily Behavioral Health

Phone: 216-252-1399

- **Address**: 14538 Grapeland Ave., Cleveland, OH 44111
- **Email**: office@dailybh.com
- **Offers**: Home-based services, school-based services, individual and family counseling, speech language services, peer social skills program
- **Website**: dailybh.com

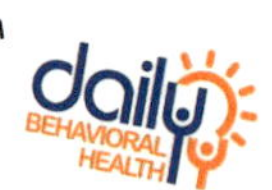

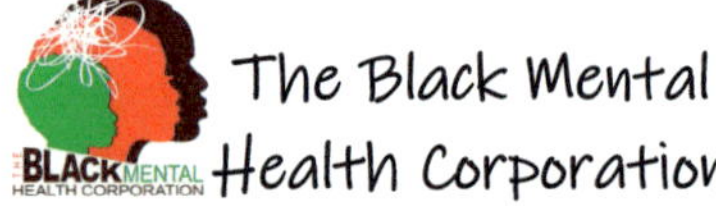

The Black Mental Health Corporation

- **Phone**: 216-512-0321
- **Address**: 13110 Shaker Square, Cleveland, OH 44120
- **Email**: helpline@tbmentalhealth.com
- **Offers**: Support groups, therapy, counseling, parenting classes, addiction treatment, social skill development
- **Website**: theblackmentalhealthcorporation.com

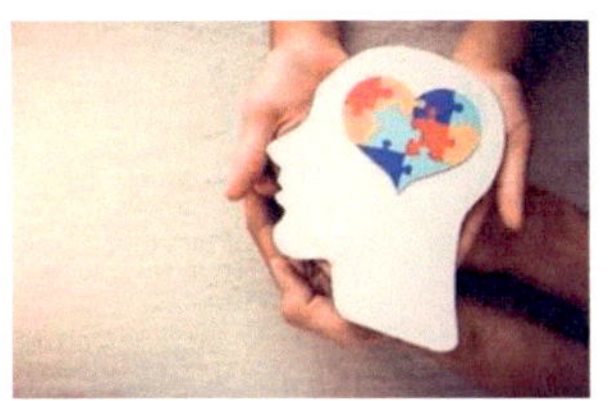

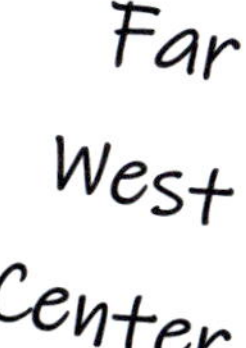

- **Phone**: 440-835-6212
- **Email**: fwc@farwestcenter.com
- **Address:** 29133 Health Campus Dr., Westlake, OH 44145
- **Offers**: Counseling, therapy, peer support, parenting programs
- **Website**: farwestcenter.com

Family Solutions

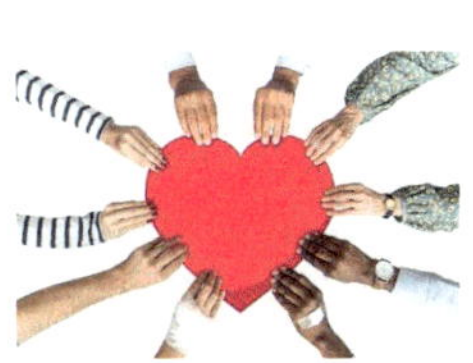

- **Phone**: 216-378-9101
- **Address**: 5198 Richmond Rd., Bedford Heights, OH 44146
- **Email:** support@familysolutionusa.com
- **Offers**: Crisis intervention, community integration, case management, outpatient treatment, crisis intervention, medication management, psychosocial rehabilitation
- **Website:** familysolutionsusa.com

Hope Behavioral Health

Hope Behavioral Health

- **Phone**: 800-642-4560 ext. 827
- **Address:** 24100 Chagrin Blvd, Ste 330, Beachwood, OH 44122
- **Messenger on Website**
- **Offers**: Counseling, therapy, spiritual care, faith-based CBT, grief services, addiction treatment
- **Website**: hopebehavioral.com

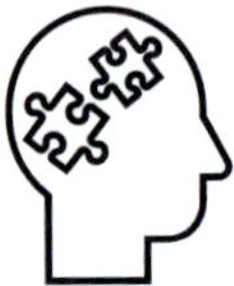

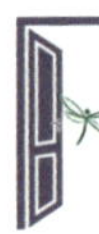

M Frierson Therapy

- **Phone**: 216-716-8696
- **Address:** 3601 Lee Road, Shaker Heights, OH 44120
- **Email**: info@mfrierson.com
- **Offers**: Psychotherapy, therapeutic/healing workshops
- **Website:** mfriersontherapy.com

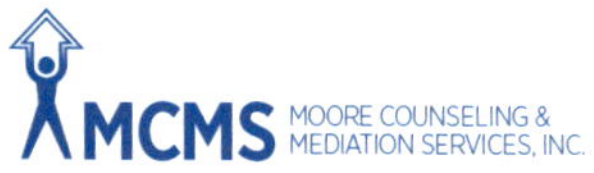

Moore Counseling and Mediation Services

- **Phone**: 216-404-1900 (Euclid Location)
- **Phone**: 216-431-4600 (Prospect Location)
- **Address**:22639 Euclid Ave., Euclid, OH 44117
- **Address**: 3622 Prospect Ave., Cleveland, OH 44115
- **Messenger on Website**
- **Offers**: Substance abuse treatment, counseling, case management, psychiatry and medication management, nurse practitioner appointments, EMDR, Equine therapy
- **Website**: moorecounseling.com

Psychiatry Networks

- **Phone**: 216-341-0070
- **Address**: 5158 Broadway Ave., Cleveland, OH 44127
- **Email**: info@psychianet.com
- **Offers**: Therapy, sleep disorder evaluations, bereavement counseling, neurological analysis and interpretation
- **Website**: psychiatrynetworks.com

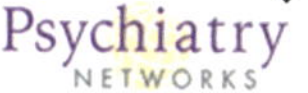

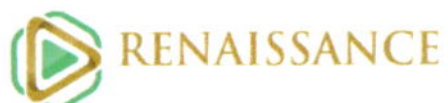

Renaissance Behavioral Health

❖ **Phone**: 440-606-2003

❖ **Address**: 3740 Euclid Ave., Ste. 101, Cleveland, OH 44115

❖ **Email**: contactus@rbhealthllc.com

❖ **Offers**: Case management, therapy, substance abuse treatment, community supportive treatment, counseling, medication management

❖ **Website**: rbhealthllc.com/

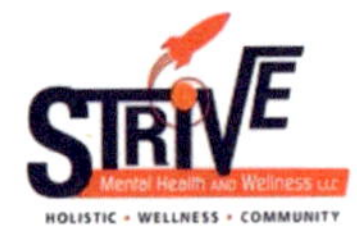

Strive Mental Health and Wellness

❖ **Phone**: 216-752-9090

❖ **Address**: 3435 Lee Rd., Shaker Heights, OH 44120

❖ **Email**: strive4today@gmail.com

❖ **Offers**: Adult mental health services, TMS treatment for depression, personalized holistic wellness plans, acupuncture, Suboxone prescriptions, wellness classes (yoga, Tai Chi, pilates, running, DJ hula hoop, boxing, TRX, drum circle)

❖ **Website**: strive4today.com

Life Enhancement Services

❖ **Phone:** 216-400-0207

❖ **Address:** 4415 Euclid Ave., Suite 335, Cleveland, OH 44103

❖ **Email:** info@lesohio.org

❖ **Offers:** mental health assessments, counseling, crisis intervention, community psychiatric support team

❖ **Website:** lesohio.org

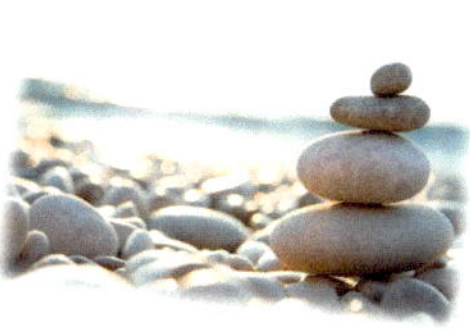

Ascend Counseling and Training Solutions

❖ **Phone:** 216-923-0333

❖ **Address:** 12200 Fairhill Rd., #A260, Cleveland, OH 44120

❖ **Messenger on website**

❖ **Offers:** individual and group counseling, case management, grief and bereavement counseling and support groups, therapeutic yoga class, consultation for school districts, training, leadership development

❖ **Website:** ascendsolutions.org

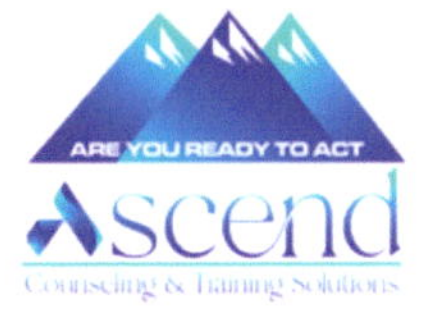

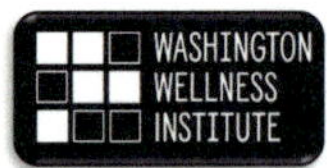

Washington Wellness Institute

- **Phone:** 216-681-9264
- **Address:** 780 E 185th St., Cleveland, OH 44119
- **Email:** info@wwillc.org
- **Offers:** counseling, therapy, intervention for family support, community mental health services, holistic and VR therapy, service workshops, hypnotherapy
- **Website:** washingtonwellnessinstitute.org

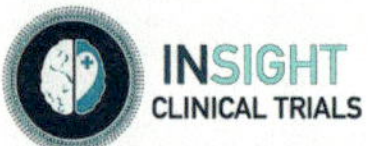

Insight Clinical Trials

- **Phone:** 216-526-1843
- **Address:** 24755 Chagrin Blvd., Suite 345, Beachwood, OH 44122
- **Messenger on Website**
- **Offers:** Phase 3 clinical trials regarding Alzheimer's, Alzheimer's with personality changes, Depression, treatment resistant Depression, Schizophrenia, PTSD, Anxiety and Depression, memory screenings, mental health consultations, offers compensation and transportation
- **Website:** insightclinicaltrials.com

Mental and Emotional Wellness Centers of Ohio

MEWCO

❖ **Phone**: 216-282-3733

❖ **Address**: 5000 Rockside Road Ste. 260, Independence, OH 44131

❖ **Email**: info@mewcohio.com

❖ **Offers**: Mental health services, virtual monthly support meetings, supervision hours, shared work environment

❖ **Website**: mewcohio.com

Serenity Health and Wellness Corporation

❖ **Phone**: 440-625-0081

❖ **Address**: 7344 Pearl Rd., Ste 2B, Middleburg Heights, OH 44130

❖ **Email**: contactshwcorps@gmail.com

❖ **Offers**: Medication assisted treatment, trauma informed care, family therapy, psychoeducation, prevention, peer support, workforce and personal development, housing, food security

❖ **Website**: shwcorps.com

Serenity
Health & Wellness Corporation

Transitioning/ Personal Development

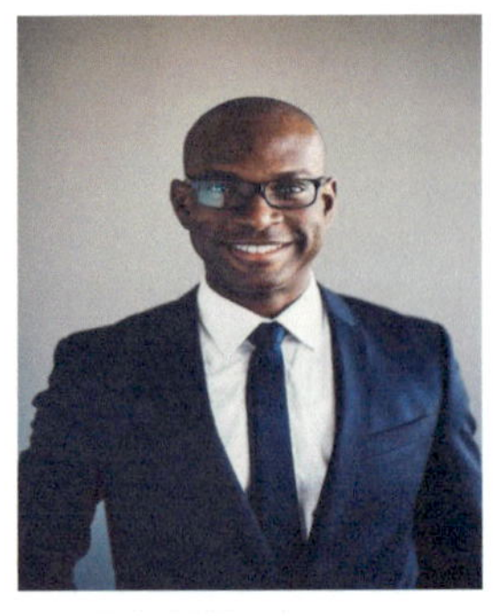

1000 Ties

- **Phone**: 216-699-0807
- **Email**: 1000ties216@gmail.com
- **Offers**: Mentorship/tutoring, Etiquette program, brand development, ages 6-21
- **Website**: 1000ties.net

100 BLACK MEN OF CLEVELAND

- **Address**: 13815 Kinsman Rd., Cleveland, OH 44120
- **Offers**: Mentorship, education (tutoring), health and wellness (awareness/education), economic empowerment
- **Website**: 100blackmencle.org

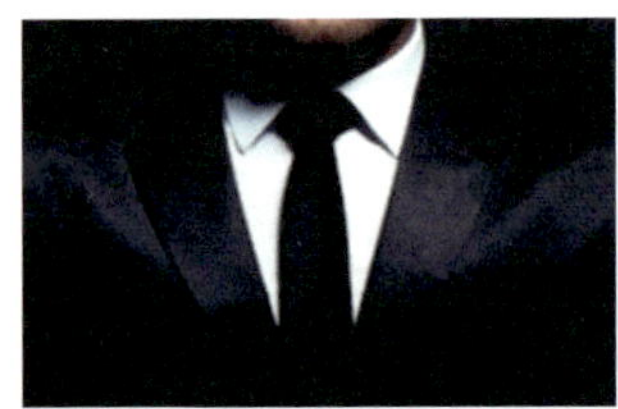

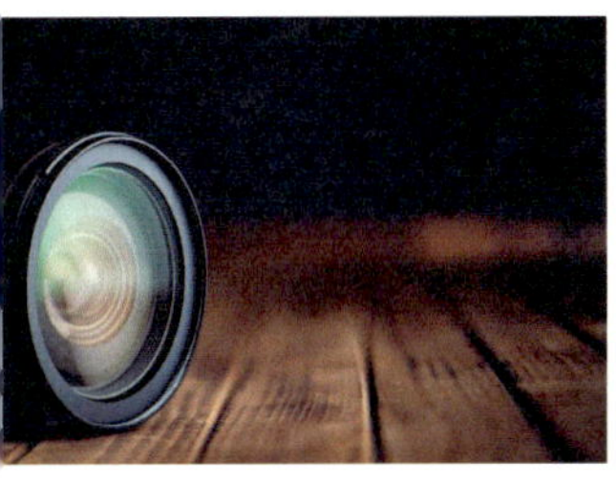

Black Space Productions

- **Phone**: 216-882-9547
- **Email**: blkspaceproductions@gmail.com
- **Offers**: Creates safe spaces for queer and trans people of color, broadcasting and media production company
- **Website**: facebook.com/blkspace/

Brandnew Community Inc.

- **Phone**: 216-404-8061
- **Email**: brandon@brandnewyouth.org
- **Offers**: Mentorship, exposure trips, community service
- **Website**: brandnewyouth.org

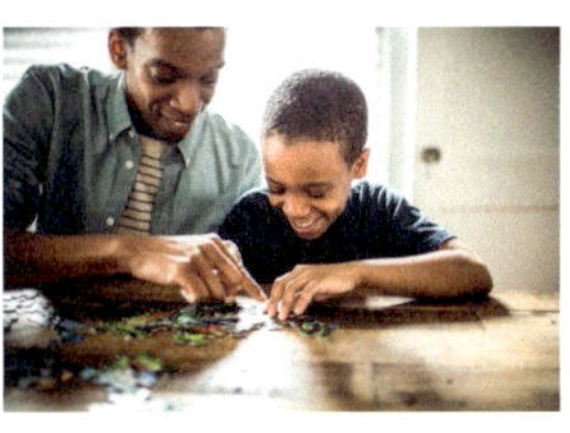

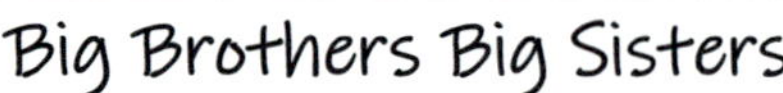

- **Phone**: 216-621-8223
- **Address**: 14837 Detroit Ave., Ste. 292, Lakewood, OH 44107
- **Email**: ttucker@bbbscle.org
- **Offers**: Mentoring
- **Website**: bbbscle.org

Boys2Men

- **Phone**: 440-539-5065
- **Address**: 487 Front St., Berea, OH 44017
- **Email**: chris@b2minc.org
- **Offers**: Mentoring, life skills development
- **Website**: b2minc.org

Broken Connections

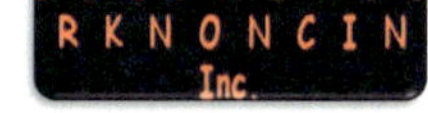

- **Phone**: 216-721-9527
- **Address**:12832 Euclid Ave., East Cleveland, OH 44112
- **Messenger on website**
- **Offers**: 24/7 on call emergency staff, shelter, clothing, food, assistance with medical care, case management, reintegration, trauma informed mental health services, linkage to community resources, life skills programming, street outreach, aftercare services for youth after they leave the program
- **Website**: brokenconnections.org

Cavaliers Community Foundation

- **Phone**: 216-420-2459
- **Address**: One Center Court, Cleveland, OH 44115
- **Email**: cavscare@cavs.com
- **Offers**: Youth sports, youth entertainment academy, Kids Club, Grant funding
- **Website**: nba.com/cavaliers/community/foundation

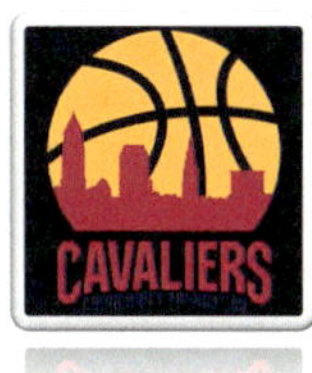

Cleveland Angels

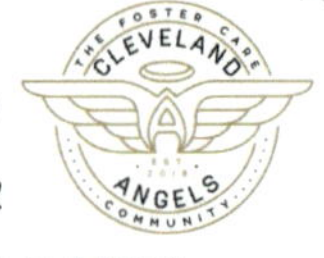

- **Phone**: 216-206-7172
- **Address**: 3615 Superior Ave. Unit 4403C Cleveland, OH 44114
- **Email**: info@cleangels.org
- **Offers**: Mentorship, support services, relationship building for children in foster care
- **Website**: cleangels.org

Community Service Alliance

- **Phone**: 216-351-0655
- **Address**: 3387 Fulton Rd., Cleveland, OH 44109
- **Email**: info@comservealliance.org
- **Offers**: Supportive housing services, career development, job placement, personal support, and life skills development
- **Website**: comservealliance.org

Distinguished Men of Excellence

- **Phone**: 216-240-4086
- **Address:** 6210 Fleet Ave., Cleveland, OH 44105
- **Email**: dme1@att.net
- **Offers**: Mentorship, education (successful transition into adulthood and responsible parenthood), volunteering, job readiness, youth empowerment groups, fitness and wellness programs, after school programs, vocational summer camp
- **Website**: dme1.org

East Cleveland Neighborhood Center

EAST CLEVELAND
NEIGHBORHOOD CENTER

- **Phone**: 216-932-3626
- **Address**: 1843 Stanwood Rd., East Cleveland, OH 44112
- **Messenger on Website**
- **Offers**: Children's Defense Fund Freedom Schools Program, HERO Elementary (STEM) Program, P.A.S.S. Program (alternative to out-of-school-suspension), social and emotional learning, Youth and Adult Mental Health First Aid, clothing and shoes for kids, substance abuse prevention, community youth diversion program
- **Website**: ecnc1986.org/

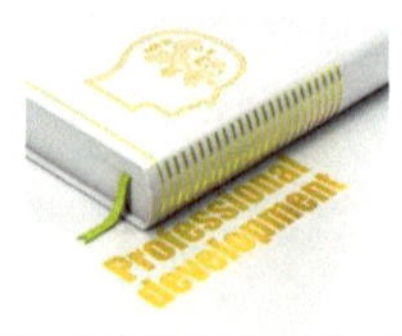

East End Neighborhood House

- **Phone:** 216-791-9378
- **Address:** 2749 Woodhill Rd., Cleveland, OH 44104
- **Email:** info@eenh.org
- **Offers:** Foster parent program, learning enrichment center, after school services, mentorship, senior center, family support services
- **Website:** eenh.org

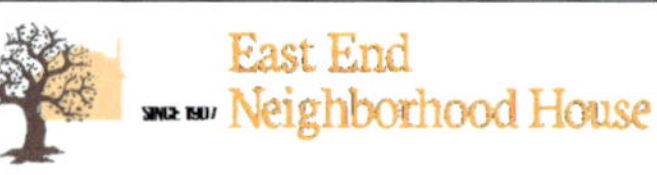

EDWINS Leadership and Restaurant Institute

- **Phone:** 216-921-3333
- **Address:** 13101 Shaker Square, Cleveland, OH 44120
- **Email:** heather@edwinsrestaurant.org
- **Offers:** Consulting, reentry program, professional development
- **Website:** edwinsrestaurant.org

Freedom Youth Program

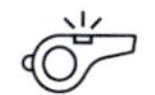

- **Phone**: 216-230-2005

Freedom Youth Program

- **Address:** 1421 East 174th Street, Cleveland, OH 44110
- **Email**: patton.z@freedomyouthprogram.com
- **Offers**: Services for young men ages 12-17, counseling, mentorship, athletic training, personal growth
- **Website**: freedomyouthprogram.com

From Me 2 U

- **Phone**: 216-307-6328
- **Address:** 13125 Shaker Square, Ste. 101, Cleveland, OH 44120

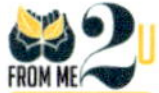

- **Email**: Lhill@fromme2uinc.org
- **Offers**: After school programming, personal development, mentorship, homework assistance, intervention programs, life coaching
- **Website**: fromme2uinc.org

Harvard Community Service Center

❖ **Phone**: 216-991-8585

❖ **Address**: 18240 Harvard Ave., Cleveland, OH 44128

❖ **Messenger on website**

❖ **Offers**: food pantry, before and after school program, summer childcare, kinship caregiver meetings, GED assistance, job readiness, parental support, housing, clothing, utility, furniture emergency services, family counseling

❖ **Website**: harvardcommunitycenter.org

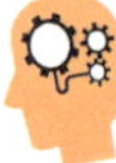

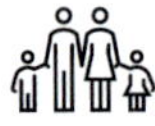

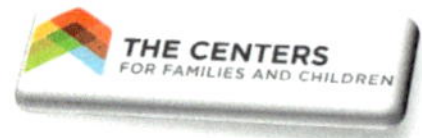

Heights Suburban Collaborative

❖ **Phone**: 216-325-9520

❖ **Address**: 1941 S. Taylor Rd., Cleveland Heights, OH 44118

❖ **Offers**: Counseling, workforce training, shoes and coat distribution, early learning, linkage to affordable housing, advocacy for families in the child welfare system, parenting classes, services for youth aged out of foster care

❖ **Website**: thecentersohio.org/services/family-support

Higher Art Life

- **Phone:** 216-618-8839
- **Address:** 7901 Central Ave. Cleveland, OH 44104
- **Email:** info@higherartlife.org
- **Offers**: Art education, teaches youth to express themselves through art, art and activism events, community programs
- **Website**: higherartlife.org

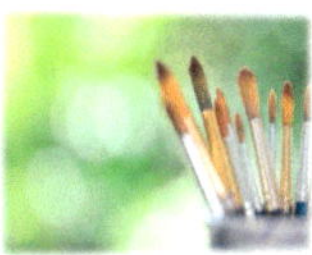

Lakewood Division of Youth

- **Phone**: 216-529-6870
- **Address:** 12525 Lake Ave., Lakewood, OH 44107
- **Email**: lakewoodareacollab@lakewoodoh.net
- **Offers**: service-learning program, community education workshops, support services for parents, families, and caregivers, juvenile diversion program,
- **Website**: lakewoodoh.gov/youth/

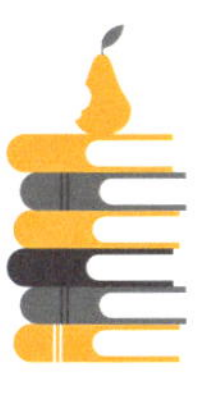

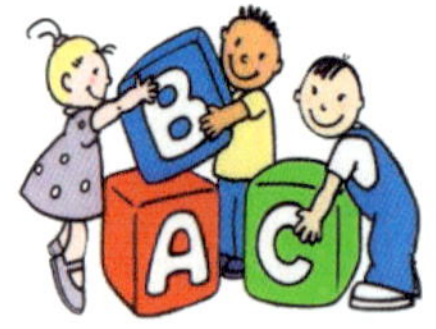

Let's Make A Change II

- **Phone**: 216-385-7770
- **Address**: 4266 Monticello Blvd., South Euclid, OH 44121
- **Email**: lmac.amc@gmail.com
- **Offers**: Childcare, housing, life skills programming, mentoring
- **Website**: letsmakeachange2.org

Learning for Life Youth Program

- **Phone**: 216-675-2223
- **Address**: 2230 Euclid Ave., Cleveland, OH 44115
- **Email**: info@ learningforlife-yp.org
- **Offers**: Mentoring, leadership programs, education development, life coaching, parenting classes, grief recovery, family retreats, arts outreach
- **Website**: learningforlife-yp.org

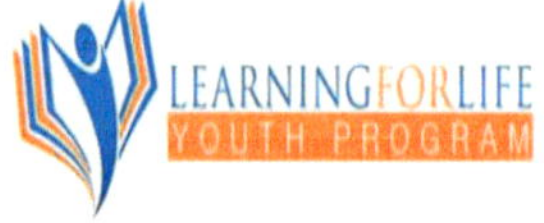

MyCom

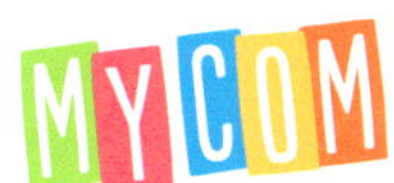

- **Phone**: 216-399-2271
- **Address:** 13815 Kinsman Rd. Suite 104, Cleveland, OH 44120
- **Email**: info@mycomcle.org
- **Offers**: Academic learning pods, youth development, youth leadership programs, Say Yes, violence and intervention program, summer learning loss prevention program, youth employment opportunities
- **Website**: mycomcle.org

National Youth Advocate Program

- **Phone**: 216-221-7588
- **Address:** 5500 S. Marginal Rd., Ste. 110 Cleveland, OH 44103

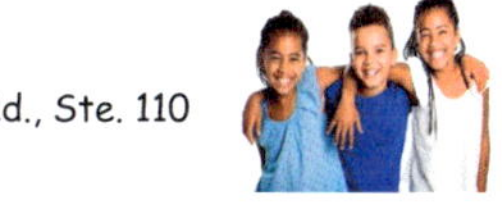

- **Offers**: Prevention and intervention, reunification, out of home placement, positive youth development, adoption, foster care, parenting education, substance use disorder treatment, workforce development, functional family therapy, intensive home-based treatment, school-based counseling, practicing alternative and safe solutions for problematic sexual behaviors

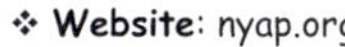

- **Website**: nyap.org

NewBridge

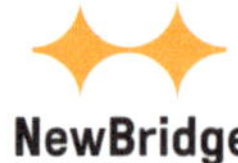

- **Phone**: 216-867-9775
- **Address:**3634 Euclid Ave., Ste. 100, Cleveland, OH 44115
- **Email**: info@newbridgecleveland.org
- **Offers**: Youth Programs, Social emotional arts-infused after-school education program, adult workforce programs (Phlebotomy Technician, Sterile Processing Technician)
- **Website**: newbridgecleveland.org

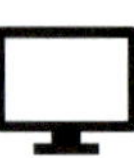

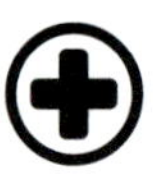

North Star Neighborhood Resource Center

- **Phone**: 216-881-5440
- **Address:** 1834 E55th. St., Cleveland, OH 44103
- **Email**: NorthStarReentry@orianahouse.org
- **Offers**: Vouchers For State Id and Birth Certificate Reentry, reunification, parenting classes, life skills classes, employment services, GED classes, computer training labs, TANF enrollment, college counseling, clothing, support groups, medical care (clinics), faith-based programming
- **Website**: northstarreentry.org

Ohio Children's Alliance

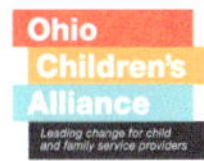

❖ **Phone**: 614-461-0014

❖ **Address:** 2600 Corporate Exchange Dr., Ste. 180, Columbus, OH 43231

❖ **Email**: admin@ohiochildrensalliance.org

❖ **Offers**: Advocacy, Bridges program, value-based care, clinically integrated health care network, Americorps, OhioReach

❖ **Website**: ohiochildrensalliance.org

Passages

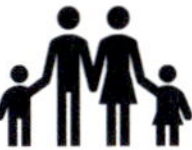

❖ **Phone**: 216-881-6776

❖ **Address:** 4600 Carnegie Ave., Cleveland, OH 44103

❖ **Email**: info@passages-oh.org

❖ **Offers:** Workforce development, parenthood enrichment services, stabilizing through employment and parenting skills program, cognitive behavioral intervention program

❖ **Website**: passages-oh.org

peel dem layers back

- **Phone**: 216-264-9794 or 216-501-1850
- **Email**: peeldemlayersback@gmail.com
- **Offers**: workshops, speaking engagements, special programs for youth and adults
- **Website**: pdlb.org

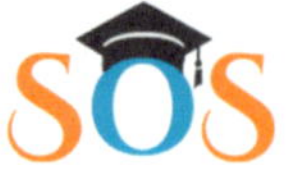

Strengthening Our Students

- **Phone**: 216-342-4381
- **Email**: sos4sustainability@gmail.com
- **Address**: 3637 Green Rd., Ste 1A, Beachwood, OH 44122
- **Offers**: life skills program, summer high school internships, after school tutoring, college scholarships, summer camp (ages 7-12), art competition project, entrepreneur education classes
- **Website**: strengtheningourstudents.com

Project Love / Values in Action

❖ **Phone**: 440-463-6205

❖ **Address**: 6700 Beta Dr., Ste. 120, Mayfield, OH 44143

❖ **Email**: abbyb@projectlove.org

❖ **Offers**: Workforce training, social skills development, character education/development programs, life skills programming

❖ **Website**: viafdn.org

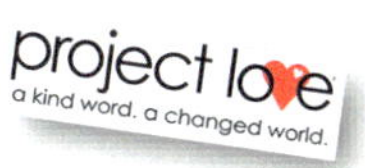

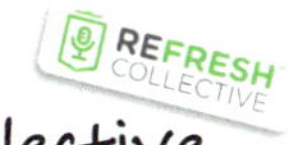

Refresh Collective

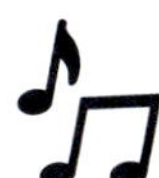

❖ **Phone**: 216-200-6373

❖ **Address**: 2800 Archwood Ave, Cleveland,OH 44109

❖ **Messenger on Website**

❖ **Offers**: Summer camp, in school programming, music making and writing as a reflective process, teaches socio-emotional intelligence,

❖ **Website**: refreshcollective.org

Renee Jones Empowerment Center

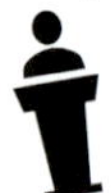

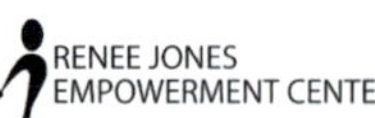

- **Phone**: 216-417-0823
- **Address:** 3764 Pearl Rd., Ste. 200, Cleveland, OH 44109
- **Messenger on Website**
- **Offers:** Therapy, tutoring, mentorship, case management, advocacy, life skills, jail and detention center visits, employment assistance, medical care, housing assistance/referrals, career readiness (interview clinics, resume assistance), youth ambassador training academy, human trafficking symposia, healthy relationship clinics, public benefits assistance
- **Website**: rjecempower.org

Shaker Heights Youth Center

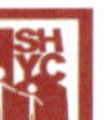

- **Phone**: 216-752-9292
- **Email**: harriet@shakerheightsyouthcenter.org
- **Address**: 3450 Lee Road, Shaker Heights, OH 44120
- **Offers**: Student assistance program (1-1, small group discussions, collaborations with parents, teachers, administrators, connects families to resources), intensive prevention program (stops school suspensions and expulsions), after school programs, hands on activities (creating outdoor furniture and playscapes for their neighborhoods), summer leadership programs
- **Website**: shakerheightsyouthcenter.org

Tamir Rice Foundation

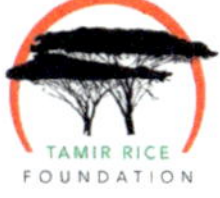

- **Address:** 6117 St. Clair Ave., Cleveland, OH 44103
- **Messenger on Website**
- **Offers:** Advocacy, after school programs for youth, speaking engagements, fundraising, community education, life skills
- **Website:** tamirericefoundation.org

Team Couture Youth Center

- **Phone**: 216-785-9244
- **Address**: 4145 Mayfield Rd., South Euclid, OH 44121
- **Email**: info.teamcouture@gmail.com
- **Offers**: Before and after school care, peer and group tutoring, summer camp, mentorship, teen power hour
- **Website**: tcyouthcenter.com

TEAM COUTURE YOUTH CENTER

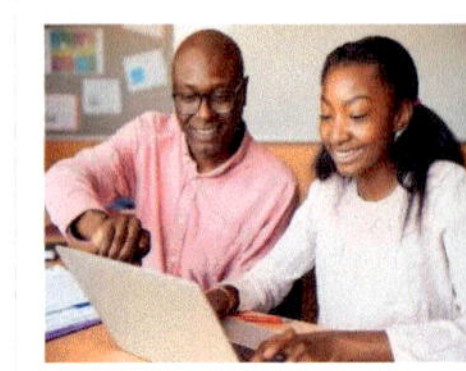

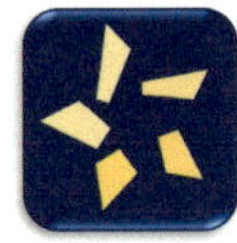

The Diversity Center of Northeast Ohio

- **Phone**: 216-752-3000
- **Address**: 3659 Green Rd., Ste. 220, Cleveland, OH 44112
- **Email**: info@diversitycenterneo.org
- **Offers**: Diversity and inclusion trainings for youth, socio-emotional learning (youth), student leadership, professional development, diversity through the arts program, adult personal development programming
- **Website**: diversitycenterneo.org

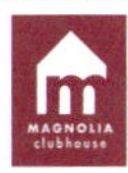

Magnolia Clubhouse

- **Phone**: 216-721-3030
- **Address:** 11101 Magnolia Dr., Cleveland, OH 44106
- **Offers:** employment and education programs, provides a safe space for people with mental illness to be social and engage with others, advocacy, social events, health and wellness dinners, daily walks, yoga and meditation, smoking cessation support, monthly health topic sessions
- **Website**: magnoliaclubhouse.org

Cleveland Hearing and Speech Center

- **Phone**: 216-231-8787
- **Address:** 6001, Euclid Ave., Cleveland, OH 44103
- **Email**: info@chsc.org
- **Offers:** Speech-language and learning, treatment for communication disorders, free online hearing screening, hearing testing, hearing aids, ASL classes, language interpreting services, vocational rehabilitation services, support services, cultural competency training
- **Website**: chsc.org

Urban League of Greater Cleveland

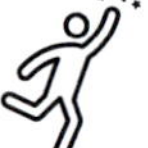

❖ **Phone**: 216-622-0999

❖ **Address:** 2930 Prospect Ave., Cleveland, OH 44115

❖ **Email**: info@ulcleveland.org

❖ **Offers:** Education and youth development (high school retention and college access program, college and university tours, MyCom), workforce development, social emotional development, entrepreneurship center, offers business loans

❖ **Website**: ulcleveland.org

See You at The Top

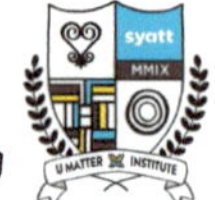

❖ **Phone**: 216-282-7448

❖ **Email**: syattcle@syattcle.org

❖ **Offers:** winter programming (skiing and snowboarding), school and community field trips, U Matter Institute (youth participatory action research and empowerment), Get Black Outside (summer programming to get youth outdoors: hiking, canoeing, kayaking, and more) consulting

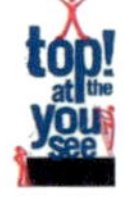

❖ **Website**: syattcle.org

Volunteers of America

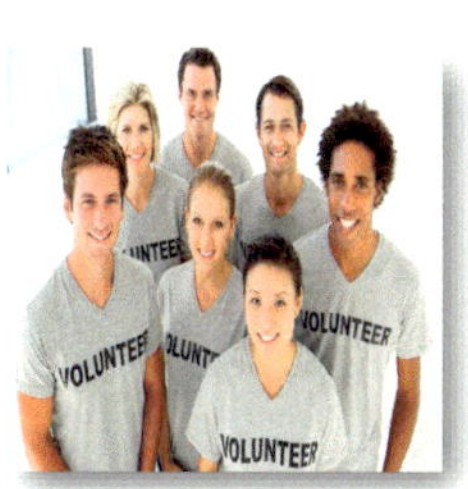

- **Phone**: 216-621-0120
- **Address:** 2710 Walton Ave., Cleveland, OH 44113
- **Email**: info@voaohin.org
- **Offers:** Veteran services, thrift stores, shelters, substance abuse treatment, parenting skills, counseling, court advocacy,
- **Website**: voaohin.org/ohio

University Hospitals Health Scholars Internship Program

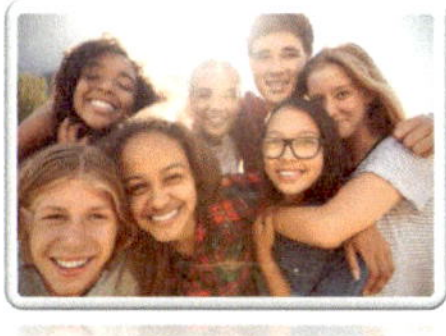

- **Phone:** 714-905-9202
- **Email**: Brittany.stone@uhhospitals.org
- **Offers:** five-year program that provides education, career exploration, leadership and professionalism development, university and medical school tours, educational field trips, opportunities to earn college credits and conduct research and network, mentoring, shadowing, weekly after school meetings, standardized test preparation, dissections and labs, journal and book clubs
- **Website**: uhhospitals.org/about-uh/diversity-and-inclusion/medical-education/health-scholars-internship-program/program-features-and-curriculum

National Alliance of Mental Illness

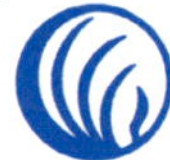

❖ **Phone**: 216-875-7776

❖ **Address:** 2012 W. 25th St. #705, Cleveland, OH 44113

❖ **Email**: helpline@namicleveland.org

❖ **Offers:** Advocacy for mental wellness and healthy transitions, support services, education, life skills programming

❖ **Website**: namigreatercleveland.org

99 Treasures Arts and Culture

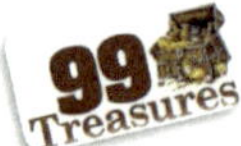

❖ **Address:** 13512 Kinsman Rd., Cleveland, OH 44120

❖ **Phone:** 216-283-5434

❖ **Email**: info@99treasures.com

❖ **Offers:** Arts programming for youth

❖ **Website**: 99treasures.org

Preventing Premature Fatherhood

❖ **Phone**: 216-201-2000 ext.1327

❖ **Email**: beaton@ccbh.net

❖ **Offers:** free educational programming focusing on healthy relationships, sexual health, consent, and exploring the role of gender

❖ **Website**: ccbh.net/premature-fatherhood

Blakk Jakk Dance Collective

❖ **Phone**: 216-468-2316

❖ **Email**: blakkjakkdanceco@gmail.com

❖ **Offer:** BJDC was created to allow dancers of color opportunities to improve their skills, perform and build a network of emerging and professional dancers. To create works of Artistic excellence and broaden the appreciation of dance in our community

❖ **Website**: blakkjakkdanceco.org

Little Giants

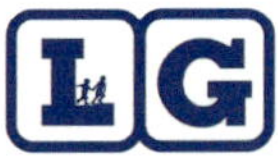

❖ **Phone**: 216-288-0527

❖ **Address:** 627 E. 185th St., Euclid, OH 44123

❖ **Messenger on Website**

❖ **Offers:** personal exercise, fitness, and wellness programs, group fitness classes, mentorships/internships, boxing academy, health screenings and assessments, fitness consultation

❖ **Website**: littlegiantscleveland.org

Thea Bowman Center

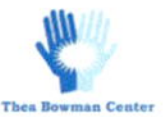

❖ **Phone**: 216-491-0699

❖ **Address:** 11901 Oakfield Ave., Cleveland, OH 44105 (On the corner of E. 120th and Union)

❖ **Email**: ella.thomas@theabowmancenter.org

❖ **Offers:** food pantry, senior outreach, GED program, online and classroom computer training, tutoring, music and Kung Fu classes, MyComm, youth summer programs, after school programs

❖ **Website**: theabowmancenter.org

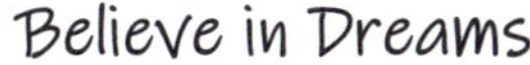

Believe in DREAMS

- **Phone**: 440-484-2376
- **Address**: 26300 Cedar Rd. Suite 1105, Beachwood, OH 44122
- **Email**: info@believeindreams.org
- **Offers**: individualized dream experience packages to empower youth towards post traumatic growth in three main areas: something they dream of learning, something they haven't had access to before, and somewhere they dream of going
- **Website**: believeindreams.org

Legal Assistance / Re-Entry

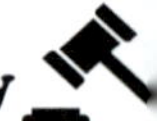

American Civil Liberties Union of Ohio

- **Phone**: 216-472-2200
- **Address**: 4506 Chester Ave., Cleveland, OH 44103
- **Email**: contact@acluohio.org
- **Offers**: internships, speaking engagements, advocacy and education around legislation
- **Website**: acluohio.org

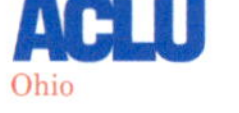

Community Corrections Program

- **Phone**: 216-781-3773
- **Address**: 1710 Prospect Ave. E, Cleveland, OH 44115
- **Email**: beau.hill@use.salvationarmy.org
- **Offers**: Reentry program, case management, Alcohol drug addiction services, housing, family emergency center
- **Website**: easternusa.salvationarmy.org/northeast-ohio/Cleveland harborlight

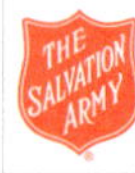

Court Community Service

- **Phone**: 216-771-2222
- **Address**: 820 West Superior Ave. Suite 310, Cleveland, OH 44113
- **Messenger on Website**
- **Offers**: Community Service, Pre-Trial Felony Diversion Program
- **Website**: ccservice.org

Cuyahoga County Office of Reentry

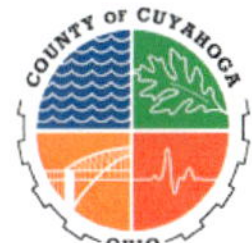

- **Phone**: 216-698-3437
- **Address**: 4261 Fulton Parkway, Cleveland, OH 44144
- **Email**: cuyahoga-reentry@jfs.ohio.gov
- **Offers**: Advocacy, community education, support services, linkage to community resources
- **Website**: hhs.cuyahogacounty.us/divisions/detail/office-of-reentry

Legal Works

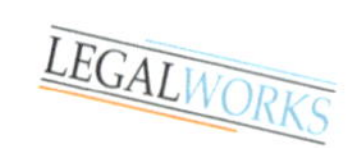

- **Phone**: 216-675-0010
- **Address**: 2800 Euclid Ave., Suite 511, Cleveland, OH 44115
- **Email**: info@legalworksneo.org
- **Offers**: Sealing and expunging criminal records, low-cost representation, restoring license privileges, removing arrest warrants, child support counseling
- **Website**: legalworksneo.org

Case Western Reserve University Milton A. Kramer Law Clinic

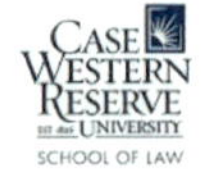

- **Phone**: 216-368-2766
- **Address**: 11075 East Boulevard, Cleveland, OH 44106
- **Messenger on Website**
- **Offers**: Appellate litigation clinic, community development clinic, criminal justice clinic (adult misdemeanor matters), First Amendment clinic, Health Law clinic, Human Trafficking law clinic, Immigration clinic, Intellectual Property Venture clinic, Second Chance reentry clinic
- **Website**: case.edu

Legal Aid Society

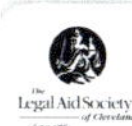

- **Phone**: 216-861-5500
- **Address**: 1223 W. 6th St., Cleveland, OH 44113
- **Messenger and applications for assistance on website**
- **Offers**: Legal Aid handles cases pertaining consumer rights, domestic violence, education, employment, family law, health, housing, foreclosure, immigration, public benefits, utilities, and tax
- **Website**: lasclev.org

CSU Cleveland-Marshall College of Law

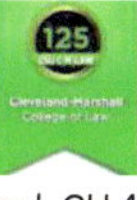

- **Phone**: 216-687-2304
- **Address**: 2121 Euclid Ave. LB138, Cleveland, OH 44115
- **Messenger and applications for assistance on website**
- **Offers**: Appellate practice clinic, civil litigation clinic, community advocacy clinic, pardon, clemency, and expungement clinic, pretrial justice clinic, transactional law clinic
- **Website**: csuohio.edu/

Education/ Tutoring/ GED/ Vocational

Allstate Hairstyling and Barber College

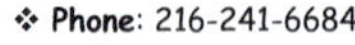

- **Phone**: 216-241-6684
- **Address**: 2546 Lorain Ave., Cleveland, OH 44113
- **Messenger on Website**
- **Offers**: Vocational barber and cosmetology training
- **Website**: allstatecollege.com

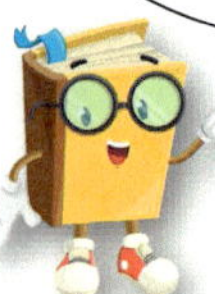

Aspire Greater Cleveland

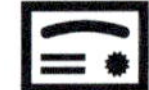

- **Phone**: 833-277-4732
- **Address**: 5225 Library Lane, Maple Heights, OH 44137
- **Email**: techols@cuyahogalibrary.org
- **Offers**: Career services, Pearson Vue testing, workplace education, tutoring
- **Website**: cuyahogalibrary.org/services/adult-education/aspire-greater-cleveland

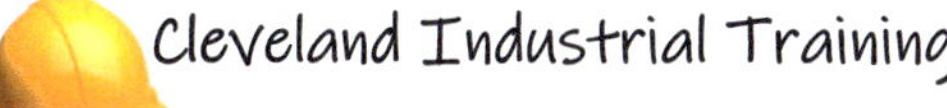

Cleveland Industrial Training

- **Phone**: 216-459-9292
- **Address**: 1311 Brookpark Rd., Cleveland, OH 44109

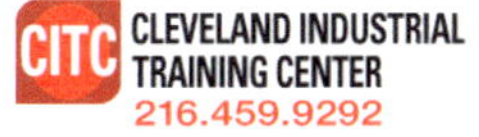

- **Email**: civery@aspraind.com or Sameer.sinha@aspraind.com
- **Offers**: Vocational training: CNC programming and operation, CNC Swiss Machine operations, job placement and pre-hire testing
- **Website**: clevelandindustrialtraining.com

College Now

- **Phone**: 216-241-5587
- **Address:**1500 W 3rd. St., Ste 125, Cleveland, OH 44113
- **Email**: info@collegenowgc.org
- **Offers**: College prep, advisors, back to school adult programming, scholarships, financial aid assistance, ACT prep, mentors, gap year program, college tours, post-secondary workshops, career technical workshops
- **Website**: collegenowgc.org

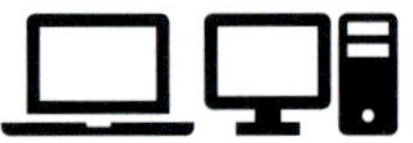

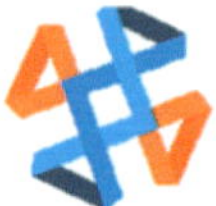

GoEngineer

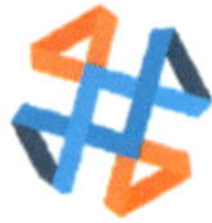

- **Phone**: 440-838-1844
- **Address**: 6060 Rockside Woods Blvd., Cleveland, OH 44131
- **Email**: info@goengineer.com
- **Offers**: Vocational IT training
- **Website**: goengineer.com/locations/cleveland

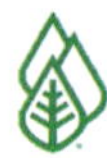

HUNTINGTON LEARNING CENTER

- **Phone**: 440-683-1784
- **Address**: 1510 Golden Gate Plaza, Mayfield Heights, OH 44124
- **Offers**: Tutoring, test prep
- **Website**: huntingtonhelps.com/center/mayfield-heights-oh

Lexington-Bell Community Center

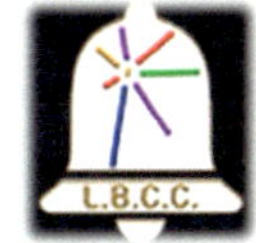

- **Phone**: 216-391-4100
- **Address:** 7724 Lexington Ave., Cleveland, OH 44103
- **Email**: lpeterslexbell@aol.com
- **Offers**: Tutoring, summer enrichment camp, early learning center, Momsfirst, Kuumba arts program
- **Website**: lexingtonbellcommunitycenter.org

Literacy in the Hood

- **Phone**: 216-469-2646
- **Email**: literacyinthehood@gmail.com
- **Offers**: Free children's books, linkage to community resources, Boys do Read program
- **Website**: literacyinthehood.com

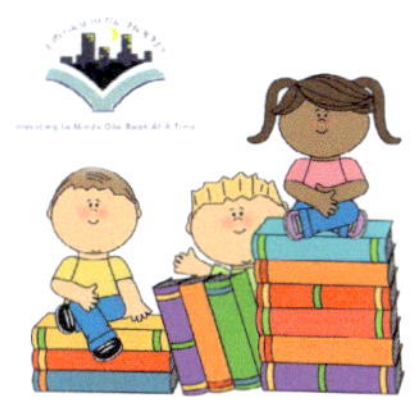

New Horizons Computer Learning Centers

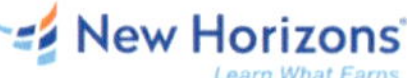

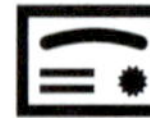

- **Phone**: 216-332-7960
- **Address**: 4500 Rockside Rd., Ste., 100, Independence, OH 44131
- **Messenger on Website**
- **Offers**: Vocational training (IT)
- **Website**: newhorizons.com

Ohio Technical College

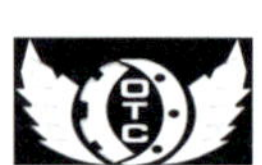

- **Phone**: 216-616-5597
- **Address**: 1374 E 51st. St., Cleveland, OH 44103
- **Email**: mambrose@ohiotech.edu
- **Offers**: Vocational training, career placement
- **Website**: ohiotech.edu

Argonaut

❖ **Phone**:
216-860-4883

❖ **Address**:
2332 Prospect Ave.,
Cleveland, OH 44115

❖ **Messenger on Website**

❖ **Offers**: American Red Cross Training and Certification, Ohio Boater Education Course, On-site Notary

❖ **Website**:
argonaut.org

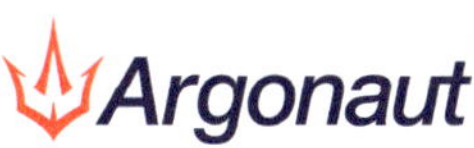

Say Yes to Education Cleveland

❖ **Phone**: 216-273-6350

❖ **Address**:
1422 Euclid Ave.,
Suite 426,
Cleveland, OH 44115

❖ **Email**: info@sayyes cleveland.org

❖ **Offers**: On-site K-12 Family Support Specialist, after-school and summer learning opportunities, mental health, pro-bono legal services, college scholarships, mentorships, connection to community resources (clothes, food, dental, medical, vision, housing)

❖ **Website**:
sayyescleveland.org

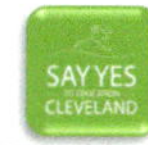

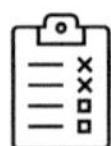

Speak into the Light

- **Phone**: 216-421-5085
- **Address:** 2490 Lee Blvd,Cleveland Heights OH 44118
- **Messenger on website**
- **Offers:** GED testing, teaches children manners and etiquette, workforce development program, First Aid/CPR/AED courses, BOSS UP business cohort (program tailored to assist entrepreneurs with building their business)
- **Website**: speakintothelight.org

Tri-C Upward Bound

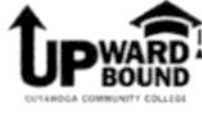

- **Phone**: 216-987-4958
- **Address:** 700 Carnegie Ave., Cleveland, OH 44115
- **Email**: christine.litvak@tri-c.edu
- **Offers:** Grades 9-12, tutoring, OGT prep and college admission test prep, assistance with college applications, 8-week bridge program for seniors, college field trips, monthly stipend, monthly Saturday seminars with guest speakers, 6 week non-residential summer program
- **Website**: tri-c.edu/trio-programs/upward-bound/index.html

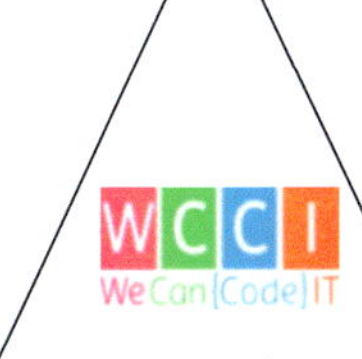

We Can Code IT

- **Phone**: 1-844-932-2626
- **Address:** 5500 S Marginal Rd., Cleveland, OH 44103
- **Email**: admissions@wecancodeit.org
- **Offers:** Vocational coding training, full time, part time, in person, and virtual options available
- **Website**: wecancodeit.org

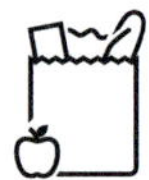

Emergency Assistance

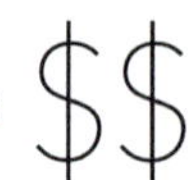

Bishop Cosgrove Center

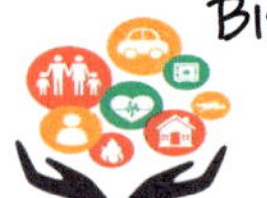

- **Phone**: 216-781-8262
- **Address**: 1736 Superior Ave., Cleveland, OH 44114
- **Email**: contactus@ccdocle.org
- **Offers**: Community meals, food pantry, emergency financial assistance, showers, identification documents, mail distribution
- **Website**: ccdocle.org/locations/bishop-william-m-cosgrove-center

Catholic Charities

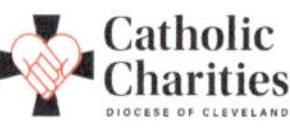

- **Phone**: 216-939-3700
- **Address**: 7911 Detroit Ave., Cleveland, OH 44102
- **Email**: contactus@ccdocle.org
- **Offers**: After school programs, assisted living and nursing care, emergency assistance, basketball, identification documents (birth certificates/ID), mail distribution, counseling
- **Website**: ccdocle.org

Cleveland Neighborhood Progress

- **Phone**: 216-830-2770
- **Address**: 11327 Shaker Blvd., Ste. 500w, Cleveland, OH 44104
- **Email**: ahalco@clevelandnp.org
- **Offers**: Financial support for communities, professional development, technical and tactical assistance to community development professionals, neighborhood economic development, workforce development, advocacy, access to capital
- **Website**: clevelandnp.org

Detroit Shoreway

- **Phone:** 216-961-4242
- **Address:** 6516 Detroit Ave., Ste. 1, Cleveland, OH 44102
- **Email:** ebischoff@nwneighborhoods.org
- **Offers:** Youth and family programming, rent and utility assistance, food assistance, income-based housing, youth leadership council, MyCom, Y.O.U., connection to resources
- **Website:** detroitshoreway.org

East Cleveland Department of Community Development

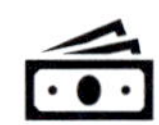

- **Phone:** 216-681-5020
- **Address:** 14340 Euclid Ave., East Cleveland, OH
- **Email:** bkyle@eastcleveland.org
- **Offers:** Emergency Assistance, unemployment assistance
- **Website:** eastcleveland.org/departments/community-development

East Cleveland Growth Association

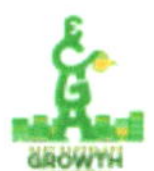

- **Phone**: 216-559-1889
- **Address**: P.O. Box 12066 East Cleveland, OH 44112
- **Email**: info@ecgrowth.org
- **Offers**: Economic development, support services
- **Website**: ecgrowth.org

May Dugan Center

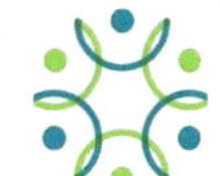

- **Phone**: 216-631-5800
- **Address**: 4115 Bridge Ave., Cleveland, OH 44113
- **Email**: amorgan@maydugancenter.org
- **Offers**: Food and clothing distribution, mental health services, education services, workforce development and placement, Moms first, senior programming, Trauma Recovery Center
- **Website**: maydugancenter.org

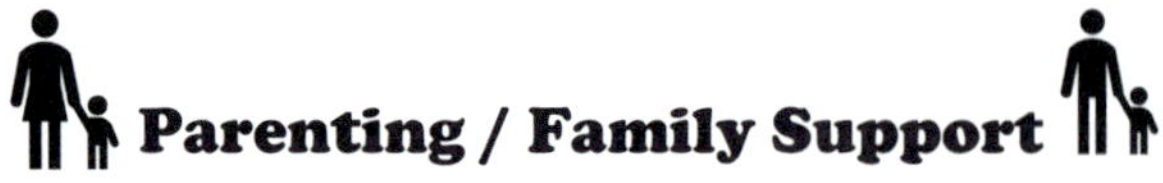

Parenting / Family Support

S.T.E.P.S – Stabilizing Through Employment and Parenting Skills

- **Phone**: 216-881-6776
- **Address**: 4600 Carnegie Ave., Cleveland, OH 44103
- **Messenger on Website**
- **Offers**: workforce development training, parenting courses, case management
- **Website**: passages-oh.org

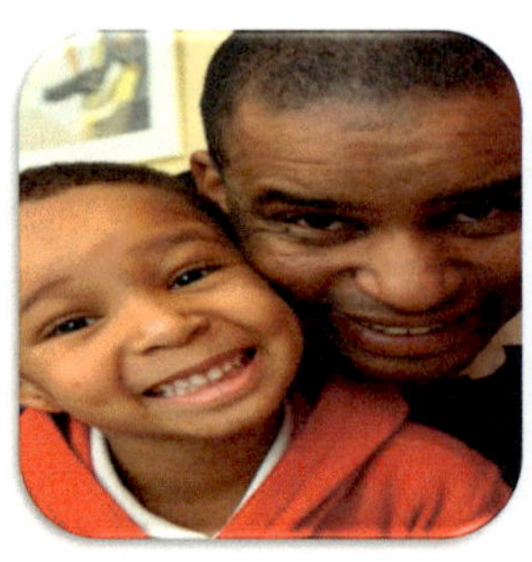

Boot Camp for New Dads

- **Address**: *There are several locations in Cuyahoga County. Locations inside Stephanie Tubbs Jones Health Center, University Hospitals, Southwest General Health Center, Hillcrest Hospital, and more*
- Contact information is listed on the website with the specific location of each Boot Camp
- **Email**: info@bcnd.org
- **Phone**: 949-754-9067
- **Offers**: Parenting classes, social support, connection to resources
- **Website**: bootcampfornewdads.org

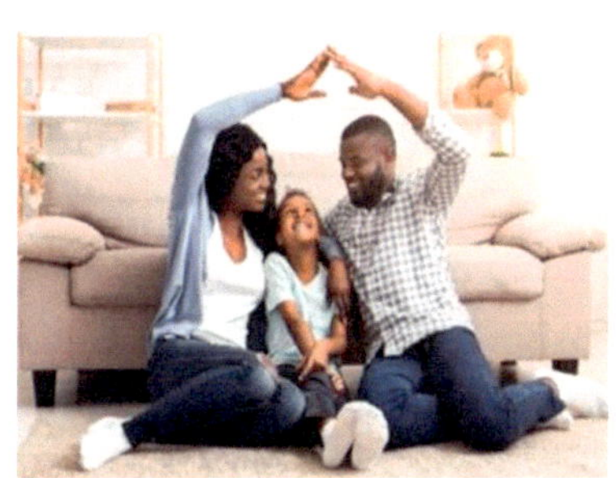

Family Connections – Shaker Family Center Facility

- **Phone**: 216-921-2023 or 216-321-0079
- **Address**: 11811 Shaker Blvd., Ste. 220, Shaker Heights, OH 44120
- **Messenger on Website**
- **Offers**: Parent support, services for children ages 0-5 years, school readiness
- **Website**:

familyconnections1.org

Family Promise

- **Phone**: 216-767-4060
- **Address**: 3470 E 152nd St., Cleveland, OH 44120
- **Offers**: Assistance finding secure housing and employment, family activities, linkage to medical and legal services, case management, temporary housing
- **Website**: familypromisecle.org

Fatherhood Initiative

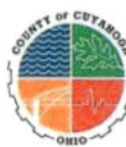

- **Phone**: 216-348-3967
- **Address:** 1640 Superior Ave., Ste. 80, Cleveland, OH 44114
- **Email**: theresa.thomas@jfs.ohio.gov
- **Offers:** Linkage to community resources (fatherhood programs, coordinated visitation, co-parenting mediation, parenting classes)
- **Website**: hhs.cuyahogacounty.us/divisions/detail/fatherhood-initiativ

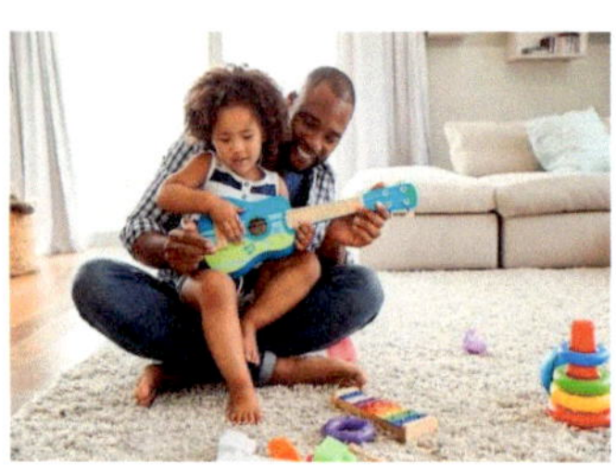

Fathers and Families Together

- **Phone**: 216-325-9124

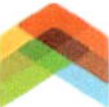

- **Address:** 6001 Woodland Ave Ste. A605., Cleveland, OH 44102
- **Offers**: Parenting classes, workforce development and training, life skills workshops (healthy relationships and parenting, community resources, legal education, nutrition information)
- **Website**: thecentersohio.org/services/family-support

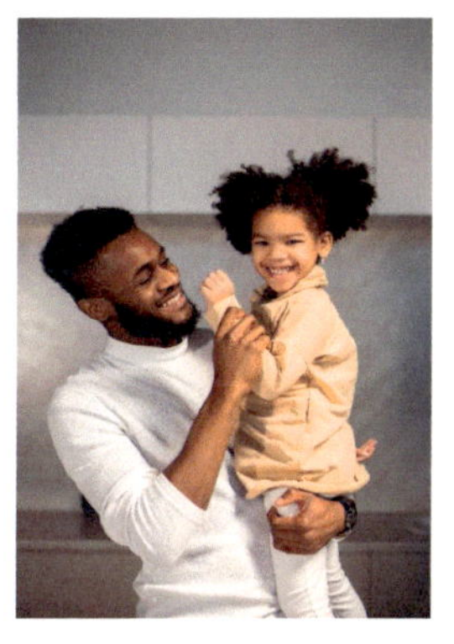

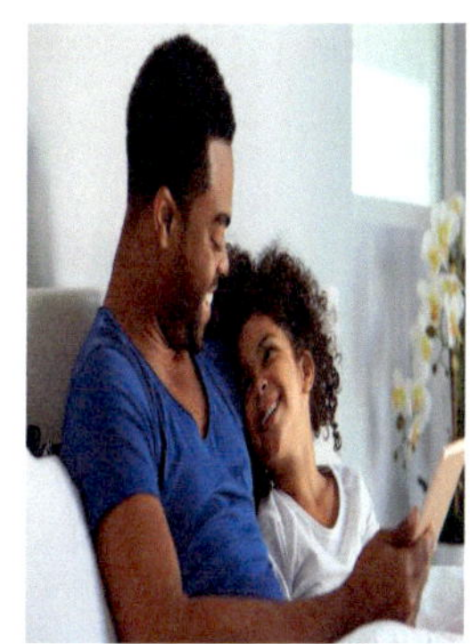

Healthy Fathering Collaborative of Greater Cleveland

- **Phone**: 216-245-7842
- **Email**: info@neofathering.net
- **Offers**: Connects fathers to resources (parenting classes, fatherhood programs, daddy boot camps, and more)
- **Website**: neofathering.net

Ohio Practitioners Network for Fathers and Children

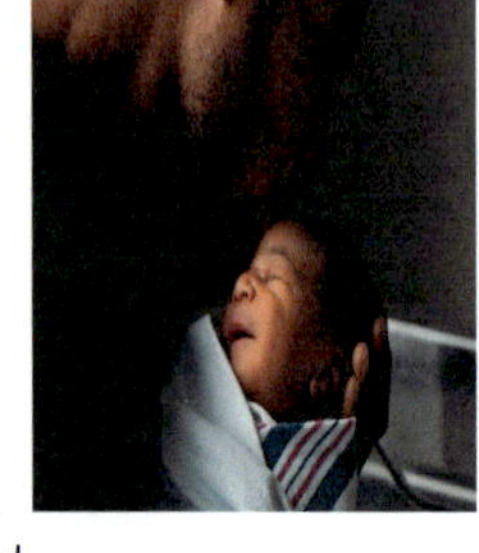

- **Phone**: 216-245-7842
- **Address:** P.O. Box 606194 Cleveland, OH 44106
- **Email**: info@opnff.net
- **Offers:** Resources for fathers (Passages, University Settlement, Beech Brook, Center for Fatherhood and Family Dynamics)
- **Website**: opnff.net

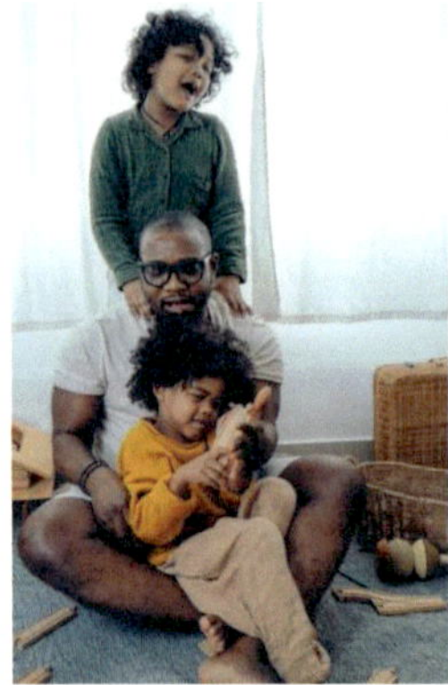

Providence House

- **Phone**: 216-651-5982
- **Address:** 2050 W 32nd St., Cleveland, OH 44113
- **Email**: info@provhouse.org
- **Offers:** Child abuse prevention, family preservation, emergency shelter, childcare, therapy, case management, parent support and classes, family trauma services, community education, community referral program
- **Website**: provhouse.org

Starting Point

- **Phone**: 216-575-0061
- **Address:** 6001 Euclid Ave., Ste. 200, Cleveland, OH 44103
- **Email**: info@starting-point.org
- **Offers:** Childcare, youth transitions program, after school, weekend, and summer programs (arts: dance, history, drama, visual arts)
- **Website**: starting-point.org

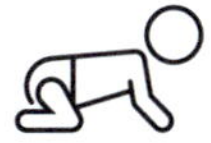

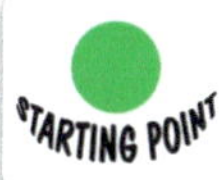

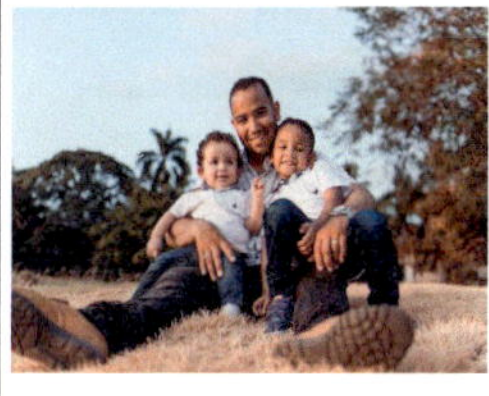

The Centers for Families and Children

- **Phone**: 216-302-3717
- **Multiple locations - check website for location closest to you**
- **Offers:** Medical care, early learning centers, home visiting, family support services, job readiness programs, job placement and supportive services, youth (18-24) cash incentives and transportation
- **Website**: thecentersohio.org

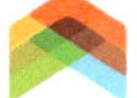

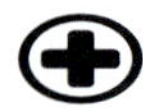 **Addiction Support** 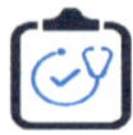

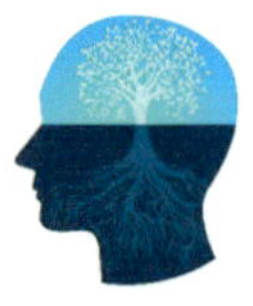

Charak Center for Health and Wellness

- **Phone**: 1-855-424-2725
- **Address**: Multiple locations: Elyria, Mentor, Garfield Heights, Medina, Stow
- **Messenger available on website**
- **Offers**: Addiction services, counseling, therapy, case management
- **Website**: charakcenter.com

Circle Health Clinic

- **Phone**: 216-325-9355
- **Multiple locations - check website**
- **Offers**: Medical care, addiction treatment, counseling, case management
- **Website**: thecentersohio.org/for/health

Highland Springs

❖ **Phone**: 216-301-2607

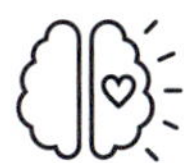

❖ **Address:** 4199 Mill Pond Dr., Highland Hills, OH 44122

❖ **Offers**: Counseling, therapy, addiction care, detox program, inpatient rehab, outpatient rehab

❖ **Website**: highlandspringshealth.com

Recovery Resources

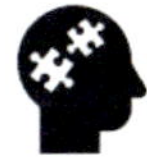

❖ **Phone**: 216-431-4131

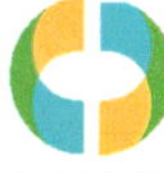

❖ **Address**: 4269 Pearl Rd., Cleveland, OH 44109

❖ **Address**: 14805 Detroit Ave., Lakewood, OH 44107

❖ **Email**: info@recres.org

❖ **Offers:** Housing assistance, prevention, employment assistance, reentry services, addiction treatment, behavioral health trainings and CEU's, recovery and support

❖ **Website**: recres.org

Saint Vincent Charity Medical Center

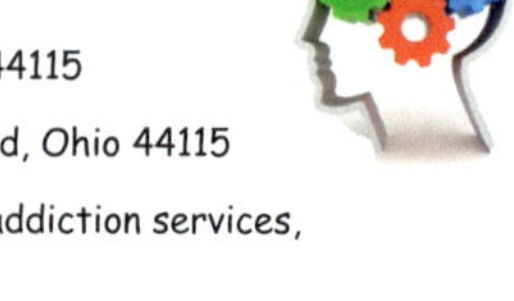

- **Phone**: 216-861-6200
- **Multiple office locations:**

  2351 E 22nd St., Cleveland, OH 44115

  2322 East 22nd Street, Cleveland, Ohio 44115
- **Offers:** Medical care, therapy, addiction services, counseling

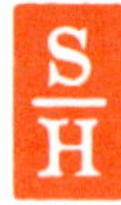

Signature Health

- **Phone**: 440-578-8200
- **Multiple locations: Beachwood, Lakewood, Maple Heights, Painesville, Willoughby, Ashtabula**
- **Offers:** Medical care, counseling, addiction services, therapy
- **Website**: signaturehealthinc.org

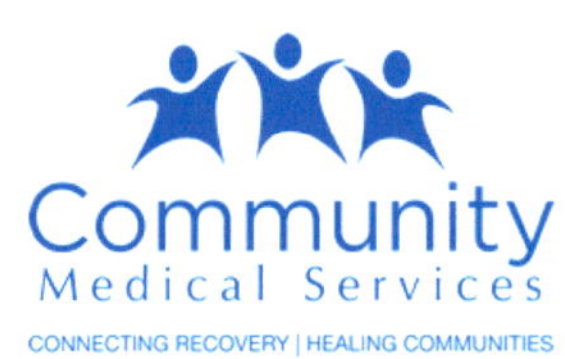

Community Medical Services

- **Phone**: 216-859-8300 Cleveland Heights
- **Phone**: 216-859-9500 Carnegie
- **Address**: 5 Severance Circle, Suite 101, Cleveland Heights, OH 44118
- **Address**: 2020 Carnegie Ave., Cleveland, OH 44115
- **Offers**: Medical care, addiction treatment and support, medication assisted treatment, individual and group counseling, correctional health services, Hep C testing, pregnancy support services
- **Website**: communitymedicalservices.org

Community Engagement

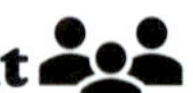

Black Empowerment Makes A Difference

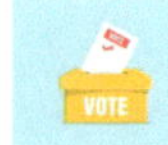

- **Phone**: 216-714-2623
- **Email**: bemad1991@gmail.com
- **Offers**: Mentoring, voter education, community activism
- **Website**: facebook.com/bemad1991

Cleveland City Council

- **Name**: Cleveland City Council
- **Phone**: 216-664-2000

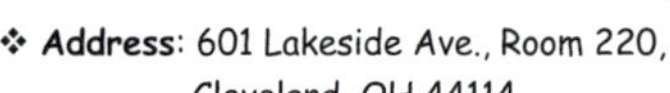

- **Address**: 601 Lakeside Ave., Room 220, Cleveland, OH 44114
- **Offers**: Monitors city departments, approves budgets, and enacts legislation to improve the quality of life in an effective and financially responsible way
- **Website**: clevelandcitycouncil.org

Economic and Community Development Institute

- **Phone:** 216-912-5655
- **Email:** clevelandreception@ecdi.org
- **Address:** 7000 Euclid Ave. Ste. 203, Cleveland, OH 44103
- **Offers:** Small business investment center
- **Website:** ecdi.org

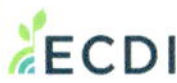

Partnership for a Safer Cleveland

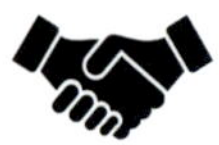

❖ **Phone**: 216-523-1128

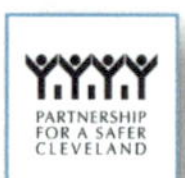

❖ **Address:** 820 W. Superior Ave., Ste. 240, Cleveland, OH 44113

❖ **Messenger on Website**

❖ **Offers:** MyCom, Police Assisted Referral, training for juvenile probation officers, youth diversion program, education and awareness, outreach and mentoring

❖ **Website**: safercleveland.org

The Center for Community Solutions

❖ **Phone**: 216-781-2944

❖ **Address:** 1300 E. 9th Street, Suite 1703, Cleveland, OH 44114

❖ **Email**: info@communitysolutions.com

❖ **Offers:** Advocacy, consulting, nonpartisan research, policy analysis

❖ **Website**: communitysolutions.com

Thrive Peer Support

❖ **Phone**: 1-877-636-3777

❖ **Address:** 29201 Aurora Rd., #400, Solon, OH 44139

❖ **Email:** info@thrivepeersupport.com

❖ **Offers:** Homeless outreach, peer support (in person, 24/7 anonymous phone support, and in hospital) support for survivors of human trafficking, support for incarcerated individuals and reentry support

❖ **Website**: thrivepeersupport.org

United Black Fund of Greater Cleveland

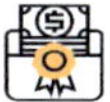

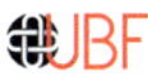

❖ **Phone**: 216-566-9263

❖ **Address:** 1621 Euclid Ave., Ste. 1200, Cleveland, OH 44115

❖ **Email**: administrative@unitedblackfund.org

❖ **Offers:** Funds community support programs: food, education, skill development (social, professional)

❖ **Website**: unitedblackfund.org

West Side Community House

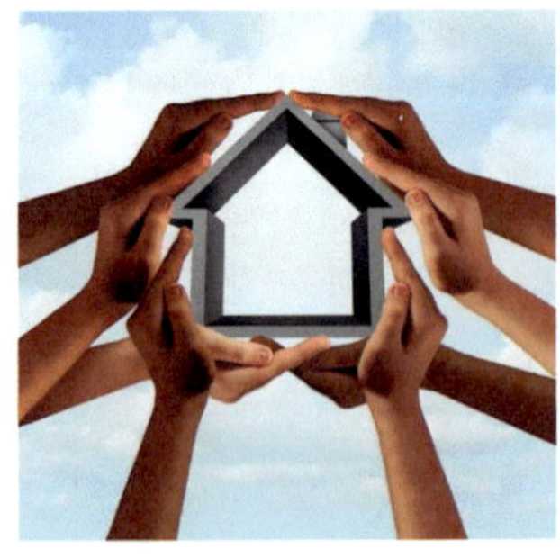

- **Phone**: 216-771-7297
- **Address:** 9300 Lorain Ave., Cleveland, OH 44102
- **Email**: info@wschouse.org
- **Offers:** Advocacy, support services, resource connection
- **Website**: wschouse.org

Westown Community Development Corporation

- **Phone**: 216-941-9262
- **Address:** 10313 Lorain Ave., Cleveland, OH 44111
- **Email**: info@westowncdc.org
- **Offers:** Community engagement, neighborhood planning, development and implementation of public benefit programs
- **Website**: westowncdc.org

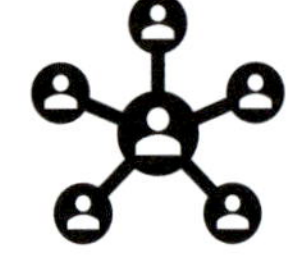

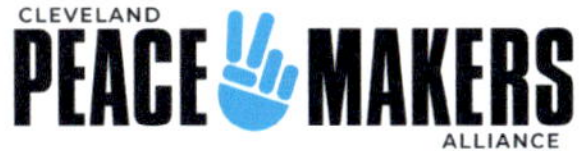

Cleveland Peacemakers Alliance

❖ **Phone**: 216-243-7002

❖ **Address:** Institute of Hope with MetroHealth Buckeye Health Center

2816 East 116th St., Cleveland, OH 44120

❖ **Email**: info@clevepeace.org

❖ **Offers:** Violence prevention, community engagement, case management, workforce assistance, safe housing, court support, safe passage, educational support, connection to community resources, hospital-based intervention following incidents

❖ **Website**: clevelandpeacemakers.org

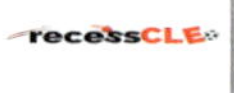

Recess Cleveland

- **Phone**: 216-242-2282
- **Email**: team@recesscleveland.com
- **Offers:** organizing games and recess at schools, community events, birthday parties, for adults and youth
- **Website**: recesscleveland.com

A Vision Of Change

- **Phone**: 216-703-2339
- **Address:** 10403 Somerset Ave. Cleveland ,OH 44108
- **Email**: avoc1993@gmail.com
- **Offers:** training and resources for Community Health Workers community health hubs, youth outreach and health summit, raising personal health awareness through education and support services
- **Website**: avisionofchange.org

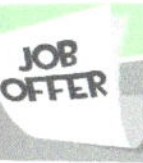

Employment Assistance

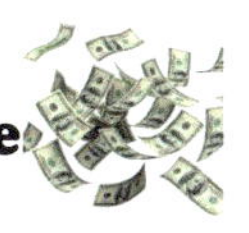

Center for Employment Opportunities

❖ **Phone:** 440-499-7131

❖ **Address:** 1500 Hamilton Ave., Cleveland, OH 44114

❖ **Email:** ceocleveland@ceoworks.org

❖ **Offers:** works with people with criminal justice involvement to reduce recidivism by providing paid employment, skills training, ongoing career support

❖ **Website:** ceoworks.org

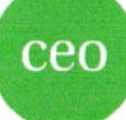

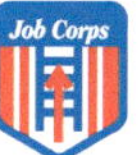

Cleveland Job Corps

❖ **Phone**: 216-541-2500

❖ **Address**: 13421 Coit Rd., Cleveland, OH 44110

❖ **Email**: Henderson.anesha@jobcorps.org

❖ **Offers**: Education, Job placement, career readiness

❖ **Website**: jobcorps.gov/center/cleveland-job-corps-center

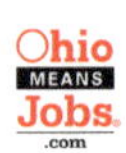

Ohio Means Jobs

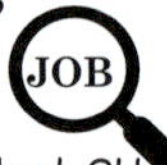

- **Phone**: 1-888-296-7541
- **Address**: 1910 Carnegie Ave., Cleveland, OH 44115
- **Messenger on Website**
- **Offers**: Job seeking, financial literacy, career fairs and workshops, practice interviews
- **Website**: ohiomeansjobs.ohio.gov/

Towards Employment

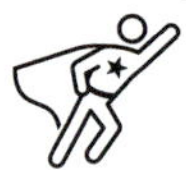

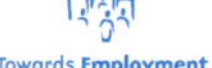

- **Phone**: 216-696-5750
- **Address**: 3301 Saint Clair Ave., Cleveland, OH 44114
- **Email**: info@towardsemployment.org
- **Offers**: Workforce development, job placement for individuals involved in the criminal justice system, legal assistance, continued career coaching
- **Website**: towardsemployment.org

Youth Opportunities Unlimited

❖ **Phone**: 216-566-5445

❖ **Address**: 1228 Euclid Ave. Ste. 200, Cleveland, OH 44115

❖ **Email**: youinfo@youthopportunities.org

Messenger on website

❖ **Offers**: Ages 14-24, leadership skills, career development, internships, support services, job placement, academic assistance, college credit plus

❖ **Website**: youthopportunities.org

Multifunction Corporations

Applewood Centers

- **Phone**: 216-459-9827
- **Address**: 3518 W 25th St., Cleveland, OH 44109
- **Email**: intake@applewoodcenters.org
- **Offers**: Counseling and therapy, case management, special needs care consultation, psychiatry, juvenile justice, foster care, residential treatment
- **Website**: applewoodcenters.org

Beech Brook

- **Phone**: 216-831-2255
- **Address**: 6001 Woodland Ave., Cleveland, OH 44104
- **Messenger on Website**
- **Offers**: Parenting classes, comprehensive sex education, therapy, counseling, anger management, supportive visitation, diversion program, homeless prevention/family stability, foster care
- **Website**: beechbrook.org

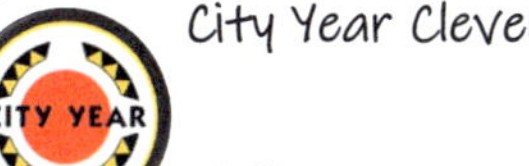

City Year Cleveland

❖ **Phone**: 216-373-3400

❖ **Address**: 3615 Superior Ave., Building 44, Ste. 44-2B, Cleveland, OH 44114

❖ **Messenger on Website**

❖ **Offers**: Life skills, education, preventative care (helps prevent dropouts)

❖ **Website**: cityyear.org/cleveland

Cleveland Foundation

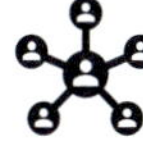

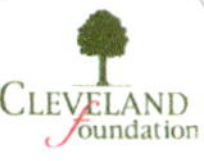

❖ **Phone**: 216-861-3810

❖ **Address**: 6601 Euclid Ave., Cleveland, OH 44103

❖ **Messenger on Website**

❖ **Offers**: Community endowment, offers grants, linkage to community resources

❖ **Website**: clevelandfoundation.org

Cleveland Metropolitan Housing Authority

❖ **Phone**: 216-348-5000

❖ **Address**: 8120 Kinsman Rd., Cleveland, OH 44104

❖ **Messenger on Website**

❖ **Offers**: Housing assistance, emergency rent assistance, housing vouchers

❖ **Website**: cmha.net

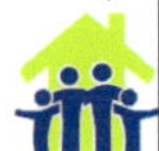

Murtis Taylor Human Services System

❖ **Phone**: 216-283-4400

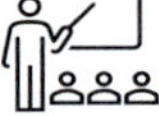

❖ **Address**: 13422 Kinsman Rd., Cleveland, OH 44120

❖ **Messenger and application for services on website**

❖ **Offers**: Early childhood education, before and after school care (tutoring), prevention, consultation, case management, foster care, information referral, clothing, computer education, parent and youth support groups, emergency financial assistance, parenting classes, fatherhood program, GED program

❖ **Website**: murtistaylor.info

OhioGuidestone

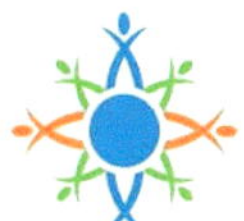

❖ **Phone**: 216-906-9568

❖ **Address:** Multiple locations

❖ **Messenger on Website**

❖ **Offers:** Counseling, residential treatment, juvenile justice programs, addiction recovery, early childhood education, foster care training and support, parenting classes and mentoring, shelters, supervised visitation, job training and employment support (in schools also)

❖ **Website**: ohioguidestone.org

YMCA

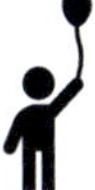

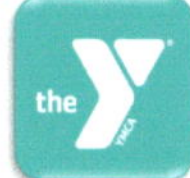

❖ **Phone**: 216-781-1337

❖ **Multiple locations**

❖ **Messenger on Website**

❖ **Offers:** Childcare, youth development programs (social skills, leadership, character), recreation center (pool, exercise, gymnasium), health and nutrition programs, temporary housing and drug treatment, re-entry program, career workforce development program

❖ **Website**: clevelandymca.org

Bellfaire JCB

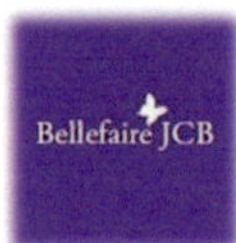

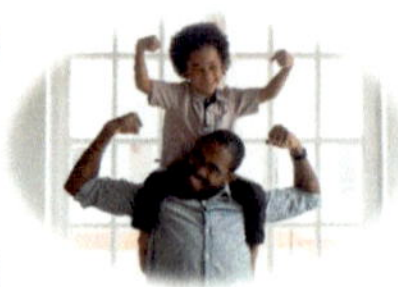

❖ **Phone**: 216-932-2800

❖ **Email**: info@bellefairejcb.org

❖ **Address**: 22001 Fairmount Blvd., Cleveland, OH 44118

❖ **Offers**: Residential treatment, counseling and therapy, autism services, adoption, foster care, early childhood education, homeless and missing youth services, prevention and early intervention, mentoring

❖ **Website**: bellefairejcb.org

LGBT Community Center of Greater Cleveland

❖ **Phone**: 216-651-5428

❖ **Email**: dastorino@lgbtcleveland.org

❖ **Address**: 6705 Detroit Ave., Cleveland, OH 44102

❖ **Offers**: health-based programs, QYou: safe and affirming place for LGBTQ+ youth ages 11-20, community resource groups, Trans and Non-binary support groups, SAGE: senior social support group for members 50 and older

❖ **Website**: lgbtcleveland.org

LGBT COMMUNITY CENTER GREATER CLEVELAND

Department of Children and Family Services

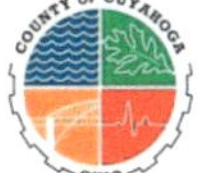

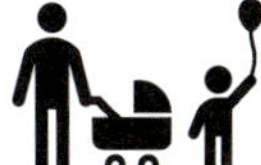

❖ **Phone:** 216-432-3334

❖ **Address:** 3955 Euclid Ave., Cleveland, OH 44115

❖ **Offers:** Resources for families and children (housing, therapy, family preservation, programs for parents, foster care, teen transitioning programs, adoption, foster care, kinship support)

❖ **Website:** hhs.cuyahogacounty.us/divisions/detail/children-and-family-services

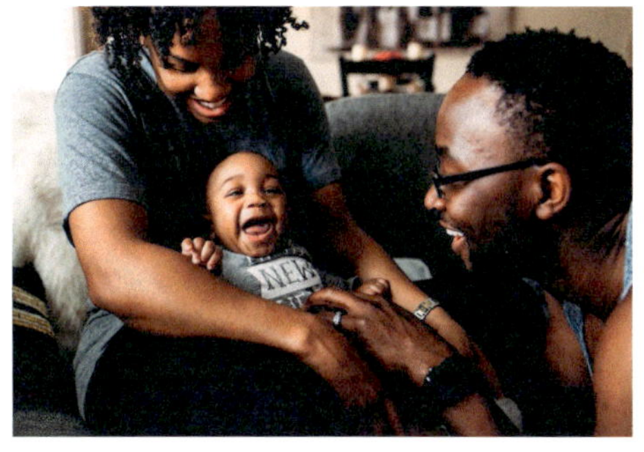

Made in the USA
Columbia, SC
07 July 2025

60169932R00064